14 Day Rapid Soup Diet

Josh

CONTENTS

14-DAY RAPID SOUP DIET

Congratulations on investing in your health and picking up the 14-Day Rapid Soup Diet!

I'm going to make this short and sweet, so you can get started with the program ASAP.

Below you'll see a 7-day meal plan.

Breakfast, lunch and dinner is all laid out for you.

Simply follow it for the next 7 days, then repeat it one more time for the entire 14-Day program.

This isn't meant to be hard.

You get to eat delicious, tasty meals every single day.

And in the process, you'll start reprograming your body to run on fat instead of sugar and carbs.

When that happens, it's only a matter of time before you lose all the weight you want.

14-Day Soup Challenge Guidelines

1. No snacking. Stick with breakfast, lunch and dinner. Eat a little more at your meals in order to hold you over to the next meal. This will get easier as your body gets used to the meal plan.

2. Get at least 12 hours between dinner and breakfast the next morning. If you finish dinner at 8 pm. Don't eat again until at least 8 am. There you go, you just fasted for 12 hours :)

3. Don't eat if you're not hungry. You never need to force yourself to eat a meal. These foods will fill you up, so if it's lunchtime and you're not hungry, don't make yourself eat. Listen to your stomach, it'll always tell you the truth.

4. Get enough salt. Your body needs salt. Especially when you cut out the processed carbs, your body will start releasing more fluids (aka water weight). With that, your body loses a lot of salt. So aim to get at least 1-2 tsp. per day. The best options are sea salt or pink Himalayan salt.

5. Before you start the program, weigh yourself and take your measurements. Use a tape measure and measure the distance around your stomach, waist, and thighs. This way you'll be able to track your progress over the next 14 days and beyond.

Approved Drinks for the Rapid Soup Diet

1. Water

2. Sparkling water

3. Lemon water

4.   Hot tea

5.   Unsweetened iced tea

6.   Coffee (no milk, sugar, sweeteners). Use 1 tsp. of heavy whipping cream or coconut oil if you'd like.

7.   Apple cider vinegar (1 tbsp. mixed with 12 oz. lukewarm water)

This plan is based on eating healthy protein, good fats, and carbs from veggies.

When you do this, it'll help lower your inflammation, blood sugar, blood pressure, and your body will start burning your stored fat for energy.

More importantly, you'll have more energy, nagging aches and pains will start to go away, your brain fog will disappear, and you'll FEEL better than you ever have before.

That's how powerful the food you eat is.

I'm glad to have you on board for the next two weeks, so... Let's get started.

Below you will see meal options for breakfast, lunch, and dinner.

Simply choose one for each meal. If you find a recipe you really like, you can make it more than once.

However, I do recommend trying all the recipes first. Then you can stick with the ones you like the best!

Breakfast (If You're Fasting, Skip These)

Chaffles (Cheese & Egg Waffles)

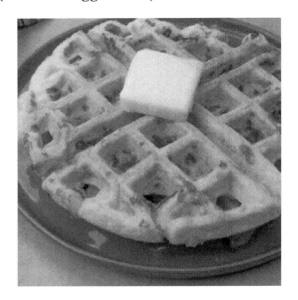

Ingredients:

- 2 eggs (beaten)
- ¼ cup shredded cheddar cheese
- 1 tbsp. butter

Directions:

1.Combine the beaten eggs and cheddar cheese

2.Pour the mixture into a warm waffle iron

3.Let it cook for 2 minutes

4.Remove and spread butter on top

Notes:

- The cook time will vary depending on your waffle maker. Usually between a minute and a half and two minutes is best.
- Shred your own cheese if possible. Store bought cheddar cheese has caking agents, chemicals, and some even have sawdust (yep, sawdust) in them. But real cheese and work your forearms shredding it yourself :)
- You can use more eggs if you like. I have a big waffle maker, so

I've done up to 4 eggs at a time in one chaffle.

Sausage, Cheese & Egg Muffins

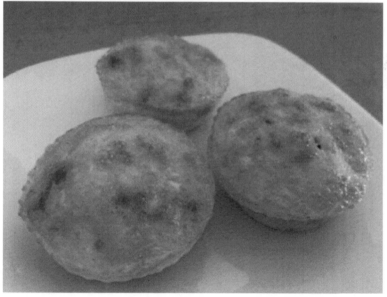

Ingredients:

- 10 eggs
- 1 cup shredded cheddar cheese

- 4 sausage links (cooked)

Directions:

1.   Preheat oven to 350 degrees

2.   Line a muffin tin with non-stick, insertable baking cups, or grease the tin with butter

3.   Chop up the cooked sausage into small pieces and add them to the muffin tins

4.   Combine the eggs and shredded cheese in a big bowl, whisk. Add salt and pepper if desired.

5.   Pour the batter on top of the sausage, evenly in the tins.

6.   Bake for 15-25 minutes, depending on the size of the muffin tin

Veggie Breakfast Casserole, servings = 4

Ingredients:

- 12 eggs

- ½ cup heavy whipping cream

- 7 oz. shredded cheese

- 1 tsp. onion powder

- 3 oz. cherry tomatoes

- 1 oz shredded parmesan cheese

- Salt and pepper

Directions:

1.   Preheat the oven to 400 degrees F

2.   Grease a baking dish with butter. Add eggs, cream, shredded cheese and onion powder to a medium sized bowl.

3.   Whisk to combine and season with salt and pepper

4.   Pour the egg mixture into the baking dish.

5.   Add tomatoes and parmesan cheese on top

6.   Bake in the oven for 30-40 minutes or until golden brown on top. Cover with a piece of aluminum foil if the casserole is getting too brown around the edges before it's cooked through

Low-Carb Granola w/ Greek Yogurt & Berries

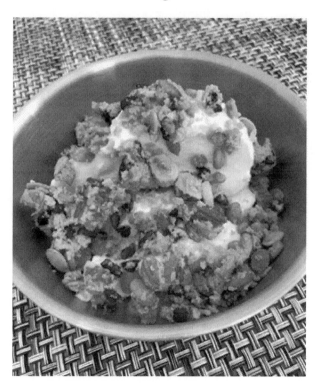

Ingredients:

- ½ cup chopped almonds
- ¼ cup sesame seeds
- ½ cup almond flour
- ¼ cup cocoa nibs
- ¼ cup unsweetened shredded coconut
- 1 tbsp. coconut oil
- 1 tsp. vanilla extract
- ¼ cup water
- 1 tsp. cinnamon

Directions:

1. Preheat oven to 300 degrees
2. Mix all the dry ingredients in a bowl
3. Heat the coconut oil, stir in the water and vanilla
4. Mix the wet and dry ingredients together
5. Line a baking sheet with parchment paper and spread the mixture evenly across the baking sheet
6. Bake for 30 minutes
7. Stir/spread around the mixture every 10 minutes so it doesn't burn
8. Serve over 1-2 cups of plain Greek yogurt
9. Add a small handful of raspberries, blackberries, or blueberries if desired.

Strawberry Coconut Cream Smoothie

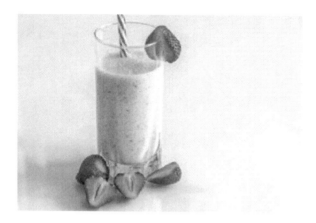

Ingredients:

- 1/2 cup coconut cream
- 2 oz. fresh strawberries
- 1 tsp. vanilla extract

Directions:

1. Mix all ingredients in a blender and enjoy!

Mushroom & Bacon Omelet

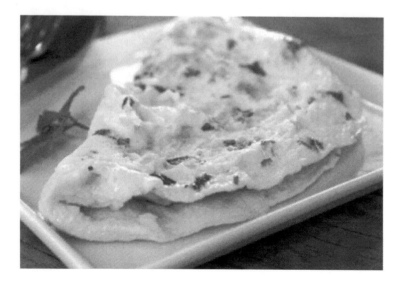

Ingredients:

- 3 eggs
- 1 tbsp. butter
- 1 oz. shredded cheese
- 2 slices cooked bacon
- 4 large mushrooms, sliced
- Salt and pepper

Directions:

1. Crack the eggs into a mixing bowl with a dash of salt and pepper. Whisk the eggs until smooth
2. Melt the butter in a frying pan. Add the mushrooms, stirring until tender, and then pour in the egg mixture.
3. When the omelet begins to cook, sprinkle cheese on top
4. Using a spatula, carefully ease around the edges of the omelet, and then fold it over in half. When it starts to turn golden brown underneath, slide the omelet onto a plate

Keto French Toast, Servings = 2 Bread:

- 1 tsp. butter
- 2 tbsp. almond flour
- 2 tbsp. coconut flour
- 1 ½ tsp baking powder
- 1 pinch salt
- 2 eggs
- 2 tbsp. heavy whipping cream

Batter:

- 2 eggs
- 2 tbsp. heavy whipping cream
- ½ tsp. ground cinnamon
- 1 pinch salt
- 2 tbsp. butter

Directions:

1. Grease a large mug or glass dish with a flat bottom with butter
2. Mix together all the dry ingredients in the mug with a fork or spoon
3. Crack in the egg and stir in the cream. Combine until smooth and
1. make sure there aren't any lumps
4. Microwave on high for 2 minutes. Check to see if the bread is done in the middle. If not, microwave for another 15 seconds
5. Let it cool and remove from the mug. Slice in half.
6. In a bowl, whisk together the eggs, cream and cinnamon with a pinch of salt.
7. Pour over the bread slices and let them get soaked. Turn them around a few times so the bread slices absorb as much of the egg mixture as possible.
8. Fry in plenty of butter and serve immediately.

Lunches

Giant Cobb Salad

Ingredients

- Spinach, romaine lettuce or salad greens mix
- 2 hardboiled eggs
- ¼ avocado
- 1-2 tbsp. Blue cheese crumbles
- 6 cherry tomatoes
- 1-2 tbsp. MCT or avocado oil
- Pink Himalayan or sea salt
- Pepper

Directions

- Combine all the ingredients to make a big salad.
- Use as much greens/salad greens mix as you like. I usually do 4-8 cups.
- For the salad dressing, pour 1-2 tbsp. of MCT oil or avocado oil on the salad, following by a generous sprinkling of sea salt and pepper

Notes:

- The amount of food you eat for lunch depends on how hungry you are. If you're really full from breakfast, don't force yourself to eat. If you're somewhat hungry, maybe you only use one hardboiled egg instead of two. Or maybe you use less cheese and avocado.

- If you're more hungry, maybe you use ½ avocado and an extra egg
- This isn't based on counting calories, so listen to your body. If you're really hungry, eat more. If you're not as hungry, eat less

Avocado Burger

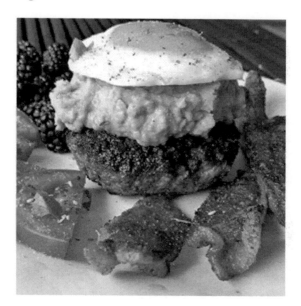

Ingredients:

- 1-2 ground beef patties
- 1-2 eggs
- ½ avocado
- Tomato

Directions:

1. Grill your burger patties
2. Fry 1-2 eggs in butter

3. Take ½ avocado and mash in a bowl
4. Place the mashed avocado on top of the burger, followed by the fried egg
5. Add other desired condiments, such as tomato, lettuce, mustard, salsa, or bacon
6. Sprinkle salt on top if desired

Fried Cabbage with Crispy Bacon

Ingredients:

- 10 oz. bacon
- 1lb green cabbage
- 2 oz. butter
- Salt and pepper

Directions:

1. Chop cabbage and bacon into small pieces
2. In a large frying pan, fry the bacon until crispy
3. Add cabbage and butter and fry until soft and golden brown. Season with salt and pepper.

Bacon, Egg & Cheese Sandwich

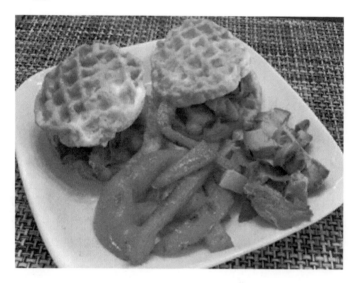

Ingredients:

- 2 eggs
- 1 oz. slice of cheese (your preference)
- 1 slice cooked bacon
- ½ avocado

Directions:

1. Using a mini-waffle maker, pour one beaten egg into the waffle maker.
2. Close and let cook for one minute
3. When it's golden brown, remove the mini-waffle and make one more. These are going to be your bread.
4. When both mini-waffles are done, make a sandwich using a slice of bacon and slice of cheese. Additional toppings

may include lettuce, tomato, or cold cuts instead of the bacon.

5. Serve with ½ avocado and veggies of your choice.

Keto Turkey Plate

Ingredients:

- 6 oz. deli turkey. Warning: most lunch meats are browned in
- vegetable or canola oil. You don't want these. Make sure to read the labels, the only ingredients should be the meat itself and maybe a few spices.
- 1 avocado sliced
- 2 oz. cheddar cheese
- 3 oz. cream cheese
- Salt and pepper

Directions:

1. Slice the cheddar cheese lengthwise, so you can wrap 1-2 slices of turkey around it.
2. Spread some cream cheese on the cheddar cheese.
3. Wrap the turkey around the cheese and eat with your hands
4. You can add the avocado to the wrap, or eat it on the side with a fork.

Fried Chicken with Broccoli and Butter, Servings = 4

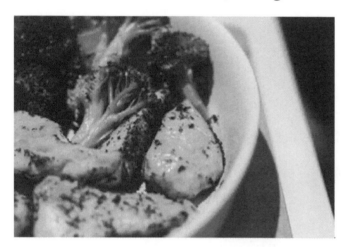

Ingredients:

- 5 oz. butter, divided
- 1 ½ pounds boneless chicken thighs
- Salt and pepper
- 1lb broccoli
- 1 tsp. garlic powder

Directions:

1. 1.Melt half the butter in a large frying pan
2. 2.Generously season th chicken with salt and pepper, then add to the pan. Flip the chicken until browned on both sides, approximately 20-25 minutes.
3. 3.Remove from pan and keep warm under aluminum foil or on low heat in the oven.

4.   4.While the chicken is cooking, rinse and trim the broccoli. Chop into bite-sized pieces.

5.   5.In a separate frying pan, melt the remaining butter and mix in the garlic powder, salt, and pepper. Add the broccoli and cook for a few minutes until it becomes tender.

6.   6.Serve the chicken and broccoli with an extra spoonful of butter melting on top

Ground Beef & Green Beans

Ingredients:

- 10 oz. ground beef
- 9 oz. fresh green beans
- 3 ½ oz. butter
- Salt and pepper

Directions:

1.   1.Heat up a frying pan with 1 tbsp. butter. Brown the ground beef until it's almost done. Add salt and pepper.

2.   2.Lower the heat, add more butter and fry the beans for 5 minutes in the same pan. Continue to stir the ground beef.

3.   3.Season beans with salt and pepper. Add in the remaining butter and cook until both the ground beef and beans are done.

Dinners

Low-Carb Turkey Soup, Servings = 4

Ingredients:

- 3 tbsp. coconut oil
- 1 yellow onion
- 1 oz. fresh ginger, grated
- 1lb ground turkey
- 1 tbsp. green curry paste
- 1 green or yellow bell pepper
- 27 oz. coconut milk
- 2 cups water
- 2 tsp. salt
- ½ tsp. pepper
- 4 oz. fresh green beans

Directions:

1. 1.Finely chop onion and ginger. Sauté in oil in a large skillet or sauce pan until onions are translucent.
2. 2.Add ground turkey and stir until fully cooked. Add curry paste and bell peppers and stir until incorporated.
3. 3.Add the remaining ingredients, except for the beans, and bring to a boil. Lower the heat and let simmer for about 20 minutes.
4. 4.Trim the beans and chop coarsely. Add to soup towards the end and cook until tender.

Low-Carb Philly Cheesesteak Soup

Serves 6

Cook time: 40 minutes

Ingredients:

- Butter – 3 tbsp.
- Green bell pepper, thinly sliced – 1
- Mushrooms, thinly sliced – 4 oz.
- Salt and pepper
- Thinly sliced deli roast beef, coarsely chopped – 1lb
- Beef broth – 4 cups
- Cream cheese, softened – 4 oz.
- Shredded white cheddar cheese – 6 oz.

Directions:

1. 1.In a large saucepan over medium heat, melt the butter. Add peppers and mushrooms, sprinkle with salt and pepper. Cook for 3-4 minutes until tender.
2. 2.Add the roast beef and mix well. Stir in the broth and bring to a simmer. Cook for 10 minutes.
3. 3.Place the cream cheese in a blender and add ¼ cup of hot broth from the pan. Blend until smooth and the cream cheese is melted. Pour the mixture back into the pan and stir in the shredded cheese until melted.
4. 4.Let cook for another 2-4 minutes, then serve.

Cream of Cauliflower with Turmeric and Pepitas Soup

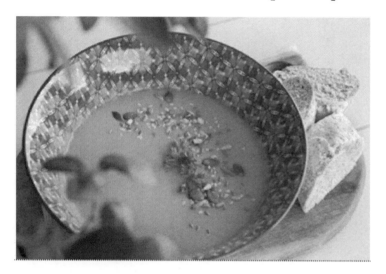

Cook and prep time: 50-60 minutes

Ingredients:

- 1 large head cauliflower, chopped
- 6 oz. full fat coconut milk
- 2 cloves garlic, diced
- 1 small spanish onion, roughly chopped
- 2 tsp. Turmeric
- 1 tsp. cumin
- 3-4 tbs. coconut oil, melted
- sea salt and pepper to taste
- 4 cups vegetable broth
- 1 tsp. Sea salt
- 1/8 cup raw pumpkin seeds (Pepitas)

Directions

1. Preheat oven to 400° F.
2. In Large bowl, blend cauliflower, oil, salt and pepper.

3. Bake on baking sheet in oven for 30 minutes.
4. Transfer cauliflower to a large pot. Add Vegetable Broth.
5. Add the rest of the ingredients, except for the pumpkin seeds, and cover while cooking on low for approximately 20 minutes.
6. Turn off heat, and using an immersion blender, blend soup until creamy.
7. Top with pumpkin seeds before serving into bowls.
8. Salt and pepper to taste.

Broccoli Cheddar Soup

Serves 6

Cook and prep time: 30 min.

Ingredients:

- Broccoli – 20 oz.
- Olive oil – 1 tbsp.
- Butter – 3 tbsp.
- Red onion, roughly chopped – 1
- Garlic cloves, chopped – 3
- Salt – ½ tsp.
- Ground black pepper – ¼ tsp.
- Paprika powder – ½ tsp.
- Cayenne pepper – 1 pinch
- Chicken broth or water – 2 cups
- Heavy whipping cream – 2/3 cup
- Cheddar cheese – 3.5 oz.

Directions:

1. Clean and cut the broccoli and separate the florets from the stalk. Roughly chop the stalks and cut the florets into small pieces.
2. Heat the olive oil with one-third of the butter in a pot or saucepan. When melted, add the chopped onion and broccoli stalks.
3. Fry on medium heat until they start to brown. Add garlic cloves.
4. Season with salt, pepper, paprika and cayenne pepper. Combine well and cook for another minute.
5. Add broth and stir well. Cover and cook for 5 minutes.
6. Transfer the cooked vegetables into a food processor and pulse. Slowly add the broth and keep mixing until you get a smooth and creamy soup.
7. In the same pot heat the rest of the butter and fry the broccoli florets.
8. Pour the blended soup mixture into the pot. Combine well and add more salt and pepper if needed. If the soup seems too thick, you can add some water.
9. Allow the mixture to come to a boil and then simmer for a few minutes.
10. Add cream and cheese and mix well. Cook until cheese has melted. Serve hot.

Hearty Mixed Vegetable Soup

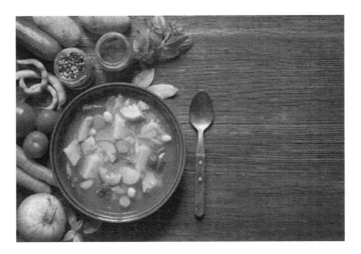

Serves 6

Prep and cook time: 1 hour

Ingredients:

- 5 Cups organic vegetable broth
- 1 cup green beans, cut in half
- 1 Medium yellow onion, diced
- 1 8 oz. can diced tomatoes in juice
- 2 Carrots sliced
- 1 Parsnip, cubed
- 2 yellow zucchini diced
- 3 cloves garlic chopped
- 2 Tbsp. Italian Herbs (basil, rosemary, oregano)
- 2 tbsp. Fresh Italian Parsley (for garnish)
- 2 Tbsp. sea salt
- 1/2 tsp. Fresh ground pepper
- 3 Tbsp. Avocado Oil

Directions:

1. In large stockpot, heat oil and add garlic, seasonings and onion. Saute for 5 minutes on low.
2. Add in remainder of vegetables with tomatoes, heat for an additional 5 minutes.
3. Add broth and cover. Simmer for 40 minutes on low, or until vegetables are tender.
4. Serve in bowls, garnish with parsley.

Italian Beefy Tomato Soup (crock-pot)

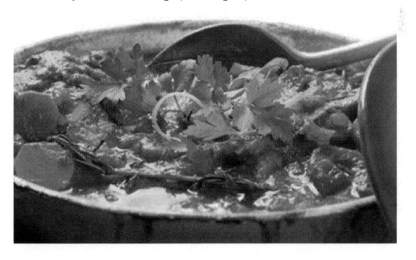

Serves 8

Cook and prep time: 15 minutes prep + 8 hours in crockpot

Ingredients

- 1 - 2 pound grass-fed beef chuck roast (pot roast)
- 3 Tbsp. apple cider vinegar
- 3 cups beef stock or broth (can use homemade, all natural or organic)
- 1 8 oz. can tomato
- 1 Tbsp. Arrowroot powder
- 3 cloves garlic diced

- 1 cup mixed mushrooms
- 2 carrots, chopped
- 1 small yellow onion sliced
- 1 tsp. dried basil
- 1 tbsp. italian parsley
- 1 1/2 tbsp. sea salt
- 1 8 oz. Can diced tomatoes in juice
- 1/2 tsp. Fresh ground pepper
- 1 large bunch of fresh italian parsley for garnish

Directions

1. Set slow cooker on low for 8 hours.
2. Add all ingredients into slow cooker except 1/2 cup of beef broth and arrowroot powder and cover. Also save fresh parsley for garnish after cooking.
3. Cook for 6 hours.
4. After 6 hours, whisk arrowroot powder with beef broth in a small bowl and blend into crock pot, stirring gently. Separate meat into large chunks with 2 forks.
5. Cook for 2 more hours.
6. Top with fresh parsley before serving.

Chilled Cucumber Yogurt Soup with Greens

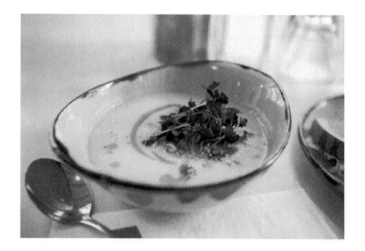

Serves 4

Prep time: 10 minutes

Ingredients:

- 2 cups pea shoots
- 2 cups, cucumbers, peeled, seeded and chopped
- 1 avocado, pitted, cut into cubes
- 1 cup plain kefir or plain greek yogurt
- 1 tsp. onion powder
- 1/2 tsp. celery salt
- 1 tbsp. avocado oil
- 1 garlic clove, diced
- Salt and pepper to taste

Directions

1. Place all ingredients from the list above in your high-speed blender, except for 1/2 of the pea shoots.
2. Blend in high speed blender or food processor until creamy.
3. Serve immediately in bowls, salt and pepper to taste, and garnish with remaining pea shoots.

KETO SOUP COOKBOOK

Just like Grandma's Classic Chicken Soup

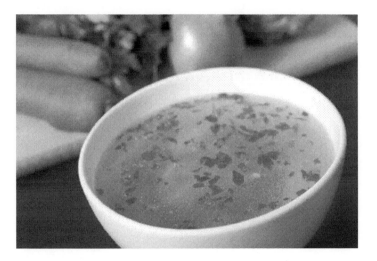

Serves 8

Cook and Prep time: 90 minutes

Ingredients

- 2 bone in chicken breasts
- 2 Tbsp. grass fed butter

- 6 cups chicken stock or broth
- 1 small onion, diced
- 2 small carrots, diced
- 2 stalks celery, diced
- 2 cloves garlic diced
- 1 tsp. onion powder
- 1 tbsp. Parsley
- Salt and Pepper to taste

Directions

1. In a large stock pot add butter, garlic, and cook while stirring for 3 minutes on medium high heat being careful garlic does not burn.
2. Add chicken to pan and cook on one side for 5 minutes, then flip and cook for 5 minutes on the other side until golden brown.
3. Add broth, and the remainder of ingredients to the pot and cover.
4. Simmer on low covered for 1 hour + 15 minutes.
5. Before serving, take out breasts, remove bones if desired and separate chicken. You can serve the broth with or without the chicken meat.
6. Serve in bowls.

Nutrition Facts Servings 6.0 Amount Per Serving calories 64

% Daily Value *

Total Fat 4 g   6 %

Saturated Fat 2 g   12 %

 Monounsaturated Fat 0 g

Polyunsaturated Fat 0 g

Trans Fat 0 g

Cholesterol 13 mg	4 %
Sodium 540 mg	23 %
Potassium 142 mg	4 %
Total Carbohydrate 3 g	1 %
Dietary Fiber 1 g	3 %

Sugars 1 g

Protein 4 g	8 %
Vitamin A	72 %
Vitamin C	4 %
Calcium	3 %
Iron	1 %

*   The Percent Daily Values are based on a 2,000 calorie diet, so your values may change depending on your calorie needs. The values here may not be 100% accurate because the recipes have not been professionally evaluated nor have they been evaluated by the U.S. FDA.

Shrimp and Bok Choy Soup

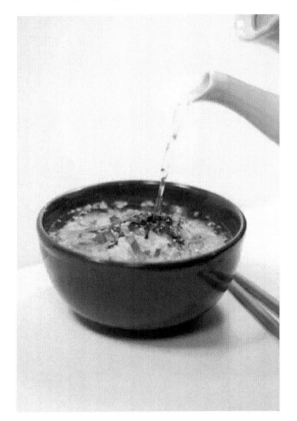

Serves 6

Prep and cook time: 35 minutes

Ingredients:

- 12 raw, deveined tail off medium shrimp
- 4 cups vegetable broth or stock
- 3 stalks bok choy, white ends cut off, chopped
- 2 stalks celery, diced
- 1 clove garlic, diced

- 2 tbsp. Butter
- 1 tbsp. Avocado oil
- 1 tsp. Sea salt

Directions:

1. In large stock pot, melt butter, oil , and add in garlic, salt, celery, and bok choy. Stir while cooking for 5 minutes on low.
2. Add shrimp, and raise heat to medium, stirring while shrimp cook for 4-5 minutes.
3. Add broth and cover. Simmer for 25 minutes on low.
4. Serve immediately in bowls.

Nutrition Facts Servings 6.0 Amount Per Serving calories 114

% Daily Value *

Total Fat 7 g   10 %

Saturated Fat 3 g   14 %

 Monounsaturated Fat 3 g

 Polyunsaturated Fat 1 g

Trans Fat 0 g

Cholesterol 93 mg   31 %

Sodium 1040 mg   43 %

Potassium 180 mg   5 %

Total Carbohydrate 4 g   1 %

Dietary Fiber 1 g	3 %
Sugars 3 g	
Protein 9 g	17 %
Vitamin A	97 %
Vitamin C	52 %
Calcium	12 %
Iron	5 %

*   The Percent Daily Values are based on a 2,000 calorie diet, so your values may change depending on your calorie needs. The values here may not be 100% accurate because the recipes have not been professionally evaluated nor have they been evaluated by the U.S. FDA.

Keto Spicy Bison Chili

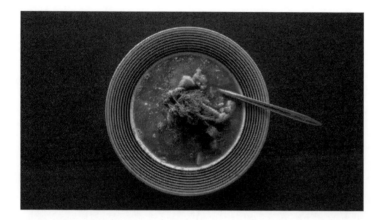

Serves 6

Prep and cook time: 55 minutes

Ingredients:

- 1 lb. ground bison
- 3 tbsp. avocado oil
- 1 medium yellow onion, diced
- 1 16 oz. can diced tomatoes in juice
- 3 cups water or vegetable broth
- 1 tbsp. cumin
- 2 tbsp. cilantro fresh or dried
- 1 tsp. cayenne pepper
- 1 tsp. chili powder
- 1 jalapeno, diced
- 2 cloves garlic, diced

Directions:

1. In large stock pot add oil, onion, garlic and seasonings. Cook over low heat while stirring for 5 minutes.
2. Add in ground bison. Stir while cooking on medium until all meat is browned.
3. Add remaining ingredients and cover. Simmer for 45 minutes.
4. Serve in bowls.

Nutrition Facts

Servings 6.0

Amount Per Serving   calories 210

% Daily Value *

Total Fat 15 g	23 %
Saturated Fat 4 g	18 %
Monounsaturated Fat 5 g	
Polyunsaturated Fat 1 g	
Trans Fat 0 g	
Cholesterol 33 mg	11 %
Sodium 99 mg	4 %
Potassium 48 mg	1 %
Total Carbohydrate 4 g	1 %
Dietary Fiber 2 g	7 %
Sugars 2 g	

Protein 16 g	33 %
Vitamin A	14 %
Vitamin C	30 %
Calcium	4 %
Iron	13 %

*   The Percent Daily Values are based on a 2,000 calorie diet, so your values may change depending on your calorie needs. The values here may not be 100% accurate because the recipes have not been professionally evaluated nor have they been evaluated by the U.S. FDA.

Spring Vegetable and Pork Soup

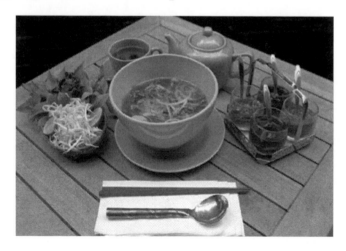

Serves 4

Prep and Cook time: 35 minutes

Ingredients:

- 12 oz. boneless pork, sliced very thin
- 2 tbsp. Sesame oil
- 4 cups vegetable broth
- 3 cups shredded cabbage
- 1 cup shitake mushrooms
- 1 spring onion, diced
- 2 cloves garlic, sliced thin
- 1 cup bean sprouts
- 3 tbsp. Fresh cilantro, chopped
- 1 tsp. Chili paste (optional to use at the end if you desire it to be spicy)
- Salt and pepper to taste.

Directions:

1. In a large stock pot, cook oil, garlic, onion and pork for 5 minutes, stirring constantly.
2. Add remaining ingredients except for chili paste, cilantro, and bean sprouts, and cover.
3. Simmer on low for 30 minutes.
4. Divide between 4 bowls. Add in sprouts, cilantro and chili paste if desired.
5. Salt and pepper to taste.

Nutrition Facts

Servings 4.0

Amount Per Serving calories 253

% Daily Value *

Total Fat 16 g   24 %

Saturated Fat 4 g   18 %

Monounsaturated Fat 3 g

Polyunsaturated Fat 3 g

Trans Fat 0 g

Cholesterol 38 mg   13 %

Sodium 757 mg   32 %

Potassium 123 mg   4 %

Total Carbohydrate 11 g   4 %

Dietary Fiber 3 g   13 %

Sugars 6 g

Protein 20 g   41 %

Vitamin A   6 %

Vitamin C   37 %

Calcium   30 %

Iron   10 %

*   The Percent Daily Values are based on a 2,000 calorie diet, so your values may change depending on your calorie needs. The values here may not be 100% accurate because the recipes have not been professionally evaluated nor have they been evaluated by the U.S. FDA.

Ground Beef and Cabbage Soup

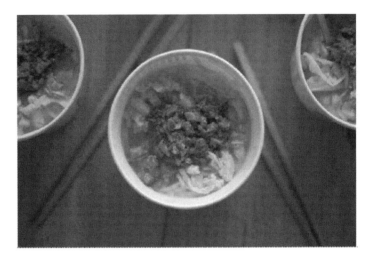

Serves 4

Prep and Cook time: 1 hour

Ingredients:

- 1 lb. ground beef
- 3 cups water, or beef broth
- 2 tbsp. Olive oil
- 2 cups green cabbage, shredded
- 1 yellow onion
- 2 carrots, peeled, diced
- 2 roma tomatoes, diced
- 1 tsp. Paprika
- 1 tsp. Apple cider vinegar
- 2 cloves garlic, diced
- 1 tsp. Sea salt
- Pepper to taste

Directions:

1. In a large stock pot, add oil, beef, onion, paprika, garlic, and salt.
2. Cook over medium heat, until beef is browned, approximately 7 minutes.
3. Add in remaining ingredients.
4. Cover and simmer on low for 45 minutes.

Nutrition Facts

Servings 4.0

Amount Per Serving calories 302

% Daily Value *

Total Fat 20 g	30 %
Saturated Fat 6 g	28 %
Monounsaturated Fat 5 g	
Polyunsaturated Fat 1 g	
Trans Fat 0 g	
Cholesterol 71 mg	24 %
Sodium 570 mg	24 %
Potassium 262 mg	7 %
Total Carbohydrate 8 g	3 %
Dietary Fiber 3 g	11 %
Sugars 3 g	
Protein 25 g	49 %

Vitamin A	112 %
Vitamin C	36 %
Calcium	11 %
Iron	19 %

*   The Percent Daily Values are based on a 2,000 calorie diet, so your values may change depending on your calorie needs. The values here may not be 100% accurate because the recipes have not been professionally evaluated nor have they been evaluated by the U.S. FDA.

Seafood Chowder

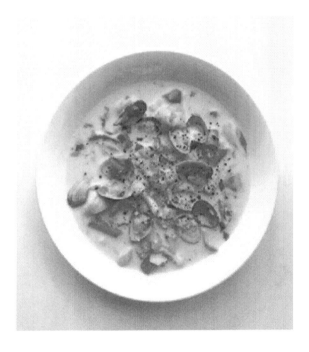

Serves 6

Prep and Cook time: 35 minutes

Ingredients:

- 12 small clams, rinsed
- 12 medium shrimp, deveined, tail off
- 2 slices bacon
- 2 tbsp. butter
- 1 cups unsweetened flax milk
- 2 cups vegetable broth
- 3 stalks celery, diced
- 1 clove garlic, diced
- 1 small yellow onion, diced
- 1 carrot, peeled, diced
- 1/2 cup heavy cream
- 1 tsp. Celery salt
- 1 tsp. Dried thyme
- Salt and pepper to taste

Directions:

In a large stock pot, melt butter, and add in potato, garlic, onion, celery, bacon and seasonings. Cook on low for 5 minutes.

Add clams and shrimp, and 1/2 cup of the broth, and cook on low, covered for 5 minutes. (clams should open up)

Add milk. Cover and cook for 10 minutes. Stirring occasionally. Add cream and continue to simmer for an additional 15 minutes. Add salt and pepper to taste after serving in bowls.

Nutrition Facts

Servings 6.0

Amount Per Serving calories 227

% Daily Value *

Total Fat 14 g	21 %
Saturated Fat 8 g	38 %
Monounsaturated Fat 4 g	
Polyunsaturated Fat 1 g	
Trans Fat 0 g	
Cholesterol 170 mg	57 %
Sodium 533 mg	22 %
Potassium 396 mg	11 %
Total Carbohydrate 4 g	1 %
Dietary Fiber 0 g	1 %
Sugars 2 g	
Protein 21 g	41 %
Vitamin A	77 %
Vitamin C	4 %
Calcium	11 %
Iron	13 %

*   The Percent Daily Values are based on a 2,000 calorie diet, so your values may change depending on your calorie needs. The values here may not be 100% accurate because the recipes have not been professionally evaluated nor have they been evaluated by the U.S. FDA.

Beef Bone Broth (slow cooker)

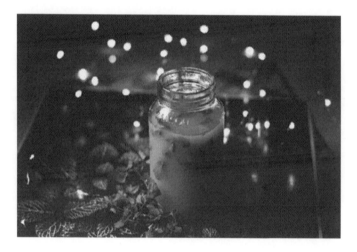

Serves 12-15

Prep and Cook time: 24 hours

Ingredients:

- 5 lbs. Beef bones. (ribs, knuckles, short ribs, oxtail and/shanks)
- 10 cups water
- 3 onions, chopped
- 1 parsnip, peeled, cut into quarters
- 3 carrots, peeled, cut in half
- 1/4 cup apple cider vinegar
- 2 cloves garlic, peeled, cut in half

- 4 stalks of celery, cut in half
- 1 cup mixed mushrooms
- 3 tbsp. Thyme
- 3 bay leaves
- 1 tbsp. Sea salt

Directions:

1. Put all ingredients into a slow cooker.
2. Set slow cooker on low and cover for 24 hours.
3. When done, remove all vegetables and bones with meat from slow cooker.
4. Shred meat off of bones, and set aside. Can use as a meal or add to other dishes.
5. Discard veggies.
6. Put broth into a large covered glass dish and refrigerate.
7. The top of the dish will get semi-hardened, and be the gelatinous part, this is the most nutrient dense part.
8. Scrape off the fat from the top heated in cups, or bowls.
9. Can freeze in small containers. Or keep in the fridge for up to 5 days.

Nutrition Facts - since most of the ingredients are discarded. The nutrient component of bone broth is approximately as follows:

75 calories

Total Carbs 1 gram

Fiber   0.3 grams

Protein   3 grams

Fat 6 grams of which Saturated   3 grams

Sodium 1104 mg

Magnesium 120 mg

Potassium 528 mg

Classic Beef Vegetable Soup

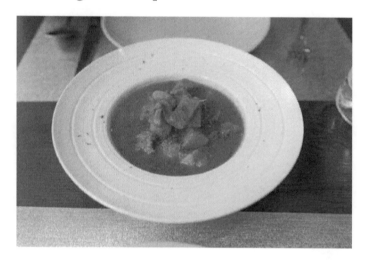

Serves 6

Prep and Cook time: 1 hour + 15 minutes

Ingredients:

- 6 Cups organic beef or vegetable broth
- 1 lb. stewing beef, cut into small chunks
- 1 Medium yellow onion, diced
- 2 cloves garlic, diced
- 1 cup green beans, cut in half
- 2 carrots, sliced
- 1 small sweet potato, diced
- 2 tsp. parsley
- 1 tsp. cumin

- 3 Tbsp. Avocado Oil
- 1 tsp. Sea salt

Directions

1. In large stock pot, add oil, garlic, seasonings and onion. Saute for 3-5 minutes on low heat.
2. Add beef, and saute for 5 minutes.
3. Add in broth, vegetables, and remaining ingredients.
4. Cover and simmer on low for 60 minutes.

Nutrition Facts

Servings 6.0

Amount Per Serving calories 233

% Daily Value *

Total Fat 16 g   25 %

Saturated Fat 4 g   20 %

Monounsaturated Fat 9 g

Polyunsaturated Fat 1 g

Trans Fat 0 g

Cholesterol 33 mg   11 %

Sodium 538 mg   22 %

Potassium 238 mg   7 %

Total Carbohydrate 8g   1 %

Dietary Fiber 3 g	5%
Sugars 2 g	
Protein 16 g	33 %
Vitamin A	75 %
Vitamin C	5 %
Calcium	9%
Iron	7 %

*   The Percent Daily Values are based on a 2,000 calorie diet, so your values may change depending on your calorie needs. The values here may not be 100% accurate because the recipes have not been professionally evaluated nor have they been evaluated by the U.S. FDA.

Chicken Stock (can use one cup of this as broth in all recipes that call for chicken broth)

Serves 12-15

Prep and Cook time: 4 hours total

Ingredients:

- 1 whole chicken, + 8 feet (feet have better flavor and minerals)
- 8 cups water
- 2 tbsp. butter
- 3 onions, chopped
- 2 parsnips, peeled, cut into quarters

- 3 carrots, peeled, cut in half
- 1/2 yellow cabbage, cut into half
- 1/8 cup apple cider vinegar
- 2 cloves garlic, peeled, cut in half
- 4 stalks of celery, cut in half
- 1 cup mixed mushrooms
- 3 tbsp. Thyme
- 3 tbsp. Fresh parsley
- 1 tsp. sage
- 2 bay leaves
- 1 tbsp. Sea salt

Directions:

1. Melt butter in a stock pot. Add in garlic, onions and seasoning. Saute for 5 minutes on low.
2. Add in all of the rest of the ingredients to the pot and cover.Simmer for 4 hours on very low heat. Skimming the foam off every 20 minutes or until broth stops foaming.
3. When done cooking. Remove all meat, bones and vegetables and use the meat, after deboning and discard the vegetables.
4. Store stock in the refrigerator or freeze in small batches for a cup of broth or a flavorful addition to meals.

**Nutrition Facts - since most of the ingredients are discarded. The nutrient component of the stock is approximately as follows:

60 calories

Total Carbs 1 gram

Fiber 0.3 grams

Protein 3 grams

Fat 6 grams of which Saturated 3 grams Sodium 1104 mg

Magnesium 120 mg

Potassium 528 mg

Beefy Onion Soup

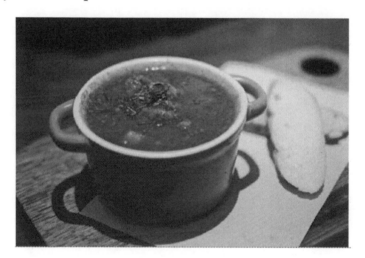

Serves 6

Prep and Cook time: 1 hour + 15 minutes

Ingredients:

- 6 Cups organic beef or vegetable broth
- 1 lb. stewing beef, cut into small chunks
- 3 Medium yellow onions, sliced thin
- 2 shallots, peeled, diced

- 2 cloves garlic, diced
- 3 Tbsp. Avocado Oil
- 1 tsp. Paprika
- 1 tsp. cumin
- 1 tsp. Sea salt

Directions

1. In large stock pot, add oil, garlic, shallots, seasonings and onion. Saute for 5 minutes on low heat until onions are soft and translucent.
2. Add beef, and saute for 5 minutes.
3. Add in broth.
4. Cover and simmer on low for 60 minutes.

Nutrition Facts

Servings 6.0

Amount Per Serving calories 195

% Daily Value *

Total Fat 11 g   17 %

Saturated Fat 3 g   13 %

Monounsaturated Fat 5 g

Polyunsaturated Fat 1 g

Trans Fat 0 g

Cholesterol 35 mg   12 %

Sodium 427 mg   18 %

Potassium 76 mg   2 %

Total Carbohydrate 4 g   1 %

Dietary Fiber 0 g   1 %

Sugars 2 g

Protein 19 g   39 %

Vitamin A   4 %

Vitamin C   1 %

Calcium   2%

Iron   10 %

*   The Percent Daily Values are based on a 2,000 calorie diet, so your values may change depending on your calorie needs. The values here may not be 100% accurate because the recipes have not been professionally evaluated nor have they been evaluated by the U.S. FDA.

Asian Vegetable Soup

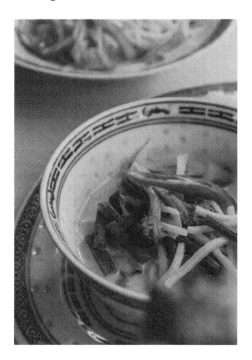

Serves 6

Prep and cook time: 35 minutes

Ingredients:

- 6 cups vegetable broth or stock
- 3 stalks bok choy, white ends cut off, chopped
- 2 stalks celery, diced
- 1 cup broccoli florets
- 1 cup shiitake mushrooms
- 1 4 oz. can bamboo shoots "matchsticks" or sliced, drained
- 1 clove garlic, diced

- 2 tbsp. Butter
- 1 tbsp. Avocado oil
- 1 tsp. Sea salt
- 1 serrano pepper, whole (optional, this will make broth VERY spicy)

Directions:

1. In large stock pot, melt butter, oil, and add in garlic, salt, and vegetables.
2. Stir while cooking for 10 minutes on low.
3. Add remaining ingredients (except for serrano pepper) and cover.
4. Simmer on low for 20 minutes, or until vegetables are tender.

Nutrition Facts

Servings 4.0

Amount Per Serving calories 138

% Daily Value *

Total Fat 9 g	15 %
Saturated Fat 4 g	20 %
Monounsaturated Fat 4 g	
Polyunsaturated Fat 1 g	
Trans Fat 0 g	
Cholesterol 15 mg	5 %
Sodium 1539 mg	64 %

Potassium 327 mg	9 %
Total Carbohydrate 12 g	4 %
Dietary Fiber Sugars 4 g	8%
Protein 3 g	6%
Vitamin A	152 %
Vitamin C	105 %
Calcium	15 %
Iron	6 %

*   The Percent Daily Values are based on a 2,000 calorie diet, so your values may change depending on your calorie needs. The values here may not be 100% accurate because the recipes have not been professionally evaluated nor have they been evaluated by the U.S. FDA.

Turkey Vegetable Soup

Serves 6

Prep and Cook time: 1 hour + 15 minutes

Ingredients

- 6 Cups organic chicken or vegetable broth
- 2 turkey legs
- 1 turkey breast, bone in, cut into 3 large pieces
- 1 Medium yellow onion diced

- 2 Carrots sliced
- 1 Zucchini diced
- 2 cloves garlic chopped
- 2 Tbsp. sage
- 3 Tbsp. Avocado Oil
- 1 tsp. Sea salt
- 3 sprigs fresh dill, chopped

Directions

1. In large stock pot, add oil, garlic, seasonings and onion. Saute for 3-5 minutes on low heat.
2. Add turkey, carrots, zucchini, and spinach, cook for 3 minutes.
3. Add in broth, and remaining ingredients.
4. Cover and simmer on very low for 60 minutes.
5. Remove turkey from pot, and with a fork and knife, remove meat from bones and add the meat back to pot.
6. Serve in bowls.

Nutrition Facts

Servings 6.0

Amount Per Serving calories 254

% Daily Value *

Total Fat 15 g   23 %

Saturated Fat 3 g   14 %

Monounsaturated Fat 5 g

Polyunsaturated Fat 1 g

Trans Fat 0 g

Cholesterol 71 mg   24 %

Sodium 1065 mg   44 %

Potassium 155 mg   4 %

Total Carbohydrate 3 g   1 %

Dietary Fiber 1 g   4 %

Sugars 2 g

Protein 24 g   47 %

Vitamin A   75 %

Vitamin C   6 %

Calcium   3%

Iron   1 %

* The Percent Daily Values are based on a 2,000 calorie diet, so your values may change depending on your calorie needs. The values here may not be 100% accurate because the recipes have not been professionally evaluated nor have they been evaluated by the U.S. FDA.

Mexican South of the Border Soup

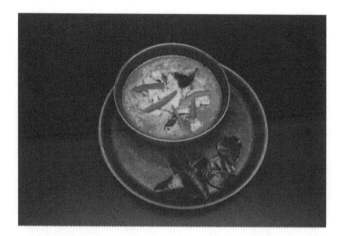

Prep and cook time: 1 hour

Ingredients:

- 2 chicken breasts, sliced into small pieces
- 3 tbsp. Avocado oil
- 6 cups chicken broth
- 1 large can petite diced tomatoes in juice
- 1 medium yellow onion, sliced
- 2 tbsp. Cumin
- 1 tsp. Cayenne pepper
- 1 tsp.sea salt
- 2 cloves garlic, chopped
- 1/4 cup fresh cilantro, chopped
- 1 red pepper, sliced
- 1 jalapenos, seeded, sliced (optional)

Directions:

1. In a large stock pot, heat oil and add garlic, onion, red pepper, jalapeno, chicken and seasonings.
2. Cook on low for 10 minutes, stirring continuously.
3. Add tomatoes with juice and cook on medium for 5 minutes.
4. Add remainder of ingredients, except cilantro.
5. Cover and simmer on low for 45 minutes.
6. Serve in bowls and top with cilantro.

Nutrition Facts

Servings 6.0

Amount Per Serving calories 155

% Daily Value *

Total Fat 8 g	12 %
Saturated Fat 1 g	4 %
Monounsaturated Fat 5 g	
Polyunsaturated Fat 1 g	
Trans Fat 0 g	
Cholesterol 15 mg	5 %
Sodium 187 mg	8 %
Potassium 251 mg	7%
Total Carbohydrate 6g	2%
Dietary Fiber 2 g	
Sugars 3 g	8 %

Protein 8 g	16 %
Vitamin A	23 %
Vitamin C	62 %
Calcium	4%
Iron	8 %

*   The Percent Daily Values are based on a 2,000 calorie diet, so your values may change depending on your calorie needs. The values here may not be 100% accurate because the recipes have not been professionally evaluated nor have they been evaluated by the U.S. FDA.

Cream of Kale, Asparagus and Broccoli Soup

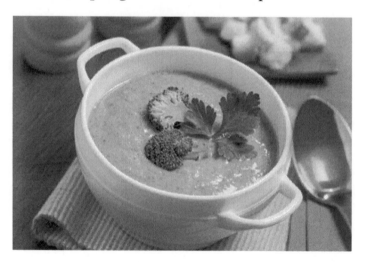

Serves 6

Cook time: 40 minutes

Ingredients

- 3 tbsp butter
- 1 small yellow onion, diced
- 2 cups broccoli florets
- 1 cup packed kale
- 2 cups of asparagus, ends trimmed, chopped
- 4 cups vegetable broth
- 1 cup full fat sour cream or 1 cup unsweetened coconut milk
- 1 tsp. Sea salt
- Pepper to taste

Directions

1. Heat the butter in a large pot and sauté onions, kale, broccoli and asparagus for about 4-5 minutes.
2. Add in broth, and salt. Cover and simmer for 20 minutes.
3. Add sour cream (or coconut milk) and simmer for an additional 5 minutes, while stirring.
4. Turn off heat, and either use a submersion blender to blend all ingredients until creamy. Or, slowly take by the cupful and add to a blender...(watch out, it will be hot!) and blend for 30 seconds in small batches, then transfer back to the pot.
5. Salt and pepper to taste.
6. Serve immediately.

Nutrition Facts

Servings 6.0

Amount Per Serving calories 155

% Daily Value *

Total Fat 12 g   19 %

Saturated Fat 8 g   41 %

Monounsaturated Fat 2 g

Polyunsaturated Fat 0 g

Trans Fat 0 g

Sodium 420 mg   18 %

Potassium 138 mg   4 %

Total Carbohydrate 6 g 2 %

Dietary Fiber 2 g   6 %

Sugars 3 g

Protein 3 g   5 %

Vitamin A   71 %

Vitamin C   15 %

Calcium   16 %

Iron   4 %

*   The Percent Daily Values are based on a 2,000 calorie diet, so your values may change depending on your calorie needs. The values here may not be 100% accurate because the recipes have not been professionally evaluated nor have they been evaluated by the U.S. FDA.

Creamy Chipotle Chicken Soup

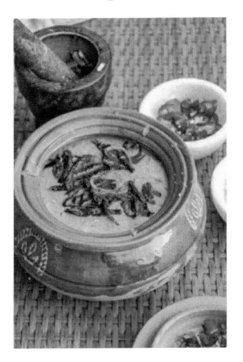

Serves 6

Prep and cook time: 1 hour

Ingredients:

- 2 chicken breasts, shredded
- 3 tbsp. Avocado oil
- 4 cups chicken broth
- 1 small yellow onion, sliced
- 2 tbsp. Cumin
- 1 tsp.sea salt
- 2 cloves garlic, chopped
- 1/4 cup fresh cilantro, chopped

- 1 small can La Costena Chipotles, sliced thin (or other jarred or canned chipotle peppers without additives)
- 1 cup plain full fat greek yogurt
- 1 red pepper, sliced
- 2 jalapenos, seeded, sliced

Directions:

1. In a large stock pot, heat oil and add garlic, onion, red pepper, chicken and seasonings.
2. Cook on low for 10 minutes, stirring continuously.
3. Add in chipotles, jalapenos and broth.
4. Cover and cook for 20 minutes on low.
5. Add in yogurt, blend and cover.
6. Cook for an additional 10 minutes on low.
7. Serve in bowls. Top with chopped cilantro.

Nutrition Facts

Servings 4.0

Amount Per Serving calories 316

% Daily Value *

Total Fat 27 g   41 %

Saturated Fat 5 g   23 %

Monounsaturated Fat 8 g

Polyunsaturated Fat 2 g

Trans Fat 0 g

Cholesterol 69 mg	23 %
Sodium 312 mg	13 %
Potassium 345 mg	10 %
Total Carbohydrate 10 g	3 %
Dietary Fiber 1 g	6 %
Sugars 4 g	
Protein 21 g	42 %
Vitamin A	31 %
Vitamin C	75 %
Calcium	15 %
Iron	17 %

*   The Percent Daily Values are based on a 2,000 calorie diet, so your values may change depending on your calorie needs. The values here may not be 100% accurate because the recipes have not been professionally evaluated nor have they been evaluated by the U.S. FDA.

Thai Vegetable Soup with Lemongrass

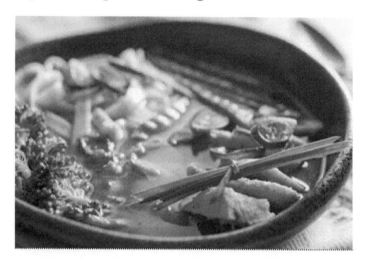

Serves 4

Cook time: 40 Minutes

Ingredients:

- 1 Tbsp coconut oil
- 2 cloves garlic, crushed
- 4 cups vegetable broth
- 10 pea pods
- 4 tbsp. Sliced red bell pepper
- Juice of one lime
- 1 tsp. Thai chili seasoning or paste
- 1 cup broccoli florets
- 1 cup mixed mushrooms
- 3 stalks of lemongrass
- 4 fresh basil leaves, chopped
- Salt & pepper to taste

Directions

1. In large stock pot, add coconut oil, garlic and all veggies except for lemongrass,and saute for 5 minutes.
2. Pour in broth. Bring to a boil and simmer for 45 minutes, covered..
3. Peel the casing off of the lemongrass stalks, and put into the pot of simmering soup.
4. Before serving, remove lemongrass stalks.
5. Salt and pepper to taste before serving.

Nutrition Facts

Servings 4.0

Amount Per Serving calories 76

% Daily Value *

Total Fat 4 g	6 %
Saturated Fat 3 g	14 %
Monounsaturated Fat 0 g	
Polyunsaturated Fat 0 g	
Trans Fat 0 g	
Cholesterol 0 mg	0 %
Sodium 243 mg	10 %
Potassium 289 mg	8 %
Total Carbohydrate 9 g	3 %
Dietary Fiber 1 g	5 %
Sugars 3 g	

Protein 2 g	4 %
Vitamin A	17 %
Vitamin C	30 %
Calcium	5 %
Iron	6 %

* The Percent Daily Values are based on a 2,000 calorie diet, so your values may change depending on your calorie needs. The values here may not be 100% accurate because the recipes have not been professionally evaluated nor have they been evaluated by the U.S. FDA.

Cream of Chicken with Scallions Soup

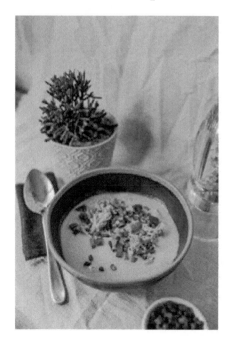

Serves 4

Prep and cook time: 45 minutes

Ingredients:

- 2 Chicken breasts, bone in
- 2 chicken thighs
- 2 tbsp. butter
- 4 cups chicken broth
- 2 scallions, chopped
- 3 tbsp. yellow onion, chopped
- 1 tsp. tarragon
- 1/2 cup full fat sour cream
- Salt and pepper to taste

Directions:

1. In a large stock pot, melt butter, add onion, tarragon, and 1/2 cup of the broth. Heat on low for 5 minutes.
2. Add chicken to the pot, cover and cook for 15 minutes on low, stirring occasionally.
3. Add remainder of the broth and cover. Cook for an additional 15 minutes.
4. Remove chicken, check for doneness. If it is not done, put back into the pot and cover. Cook for an additional 5 minutes.
5. Remove chicken, shred meat from bones, discard bones and add meat back to the pot.
6. Add sour cream and stir slowly while simmering on low for 3-5 minutes.
7. Serve in bowls.

Nutrition Facts

Servings 4.0

Amount Per Serving calories 197

% Daily Value *

Total Fat 11 g	16 %
Saturated Fat 5 g	25 %
Monounsaturated Fat 3 g	
Polyunsaturated Fat 1 g	
Trans Fat 0 g	
Cholesterol 60 mg	20 %
Sodium 234 mg	10 %
Potassium 183 mg	5 %
Total Carbohydrate 3 g	1 %
Dietary Fiber 1 g	3 %
Sugars 1 g	
Protein 15 g	30 %
Vitamin A	54 %
Vitamin C	11 %
Calcium	6 %
Iron	5 %

*   The Percent Daily Values are based on a 2,000 calorie diet, so your values may change depending on your calorie needs. The values here may not be 100% accurate because the recipes have not been professionally evaluated nor have they been evaluated by the U.S. FDA.

Chicken Cilantro and Lime Soup

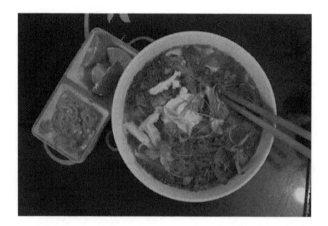

Serves 6

Cook and Prep time: 90 minutes

Ingredients

- 2 chicken breast fillets, torn by hand into small pieces
- 2 Tbsp. sesame oil
- 6 cups chicken stock or broth
- 1 small onion, diced
- 1 cup cilantro
- 2 stalks celery, diced
- 2 cloves garlic diced
- 1 tsp. onion powder
- 1 tbsp. Parsley
- Juice of one lime
- Salt and Pepper to taste

Directions

1. In a large stock pot add oil, garlic, and cook while stirring for 3 minutes on medium high heat being careful garlic does not burn.
2. Add chicken to pan, and remaining ingredients and cook while stirring for 10 minutes on low .
3. Add broth to the pot and cover.
4. Simmer on low covered for 45 minutes.
5. Serve in bowls.

Nutrition Facts

Servings 6.0

Amount Per Serving calories 164

% Daily Value *

Total Fat 6 g	10 %
Saturated Fat 1 g	6 %
Monounsaturated Fat 2 g	
Polyunsaturated Fat 2 g	
Trans Fat 0 g	
Cholesterol 89 mg	30 %
Sodium 304 mg	13 %
Potassium 73 mg	2%
Total Carbohydrate 5g	2 %
Dietary Fiber 1g	3%
Sugars 1 g	

Protein 22 g   43 %

Vitamin A   25 %

Vitamin C   18 %

Calcium   6%

Iron   7 %

*   The Percent Daily Values are based on a 2,000 calorie diet, so your values may change depending on your calorie needs. The values here may not be 100% accurate because the recipes have not been professionally evaluated nor have they been evaluated by the U.S. FDA.

Cream of Asparagus and Cauliflower Soup

Serves 4

Cook time: 40 minutes

Ingredients

- 3 tbsp butter
- 1 small yellow onion, diced
- 2 celery stalks, chopped
- 2 cloves garlic, diced
- 1/2 head cauliflower, chopped
- 2 cups asparagus stalks, trimmed and chopped
- 3 cups vegetable broth
- 1 cup unsweetened coconut or almond milk
- 1 tsp. Sea salt

- Pepper to taste

Directions

1. Heat the butter in a large pot on low, and sauté onion, celery, garlic, cauliflower and asparagus and for about 10 minutes.
2. Add in broth, and salt. Cover and simmer for 20 minutes.
3. Add coconut milk and simmer for an additional 5 minutes, while stirring.
4. Turn off heat, and either use a submersion blender to blend all ingredients until creamy. Or, slowly take by the cupful and add to a blender...(watch out, it will be hot!)
5. Blend for 30 seconds then transfer back to the pot.
6. Serve immediately.

Nutrition Facts

Servings 4.0

Amount Per Serving calories 107

% Daily Value *

Total Fat 10 g   15 %

Saturated Fat 6 g   32 %

Monounsaturated Fat 2 g

Polyunsaturated Fat 0 g

Trans Fat 0 g

Cholesterol 23 mg   8 %

Sodium 608 mg	25 %
Potassium 151 mg	4 %
Total Carbohydrate 6 g	2 %
Dietary Fiber 3 g	5 %
Sugars 2 g	
Protein 1 g	1 %
Vitamin A	80 %
Vitamin C	3 %
Calcium	19 %
Iron	4 %

*   The Percent Daily Values are based on a 2,000 calorie diet, so your values may change depending on your calorie needs. The values here may not be 100% accurate because the recipes have not been professionally evaluated nor have they been evaluated by the U.S. FDA.

Spices of India Curried Vegetable Soup

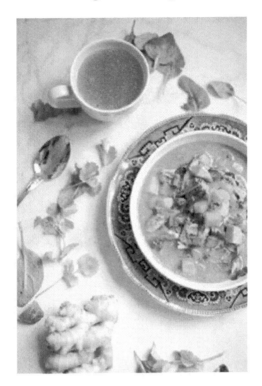

Serves 6

Prep and Cook time: 1 hour

Ingredients:

- 3 tbsp. Ghee
- 1 sweet potato, peeled, cut into cubes
- 1 cup butternut squash, peeled, cubed
- 1 small onion, diced
- 2 cloves garlic, diced
- 1 8oz. Can full fat coconut milk
- 4 tbsp. Fresh Cilantro (for garnish)
- 1 tbsp. Turmeric
- 1 tsp. Curry masala seasoning

- 1 tsp. Ginger powder, or root peeled and diced
- 3 cups vegetable broth
- 1 tsp salt
- Pepper to taste

Directions:

1. In a large stock pot, melt ghee on low and add salt, garlic, onions, potatoes, squash, and seasonings. Cook for 5 minutes.
2. Add in broth, and cover. Cook for 30 minutes or until potatoes are tender.
3. Add in coconut milk. Stir and cover for 10 minutes.
4. Serve in bowls topped with chopped cilantro.

Nutrition Facts

Servings 6.0

Amount Per Serving calories 233

% Daily Value *

Total Fat 20 g   30 %

Saturated Fat 14 g   70 %

Monounsaturated Fat 1 g

Polyunsaturated Fat 0 g

Trans Fat 0 g

Cholesterol 0 mg   0 %

Sodium 499 mg   21 %

Potassium 245 mg   7 %

Total Carbohydrate 15 g	5 %
Dietary Fiber 2 g	7%
Sugars 4g	
Protein 1 g	2%
Vitamin A	163 %
Vitamin C	19 %
Calcium	5 %
Iron	8 %

*   The Percent Daily Values are based on a 2,000 calorie diet, so your values may change depending on your calorie needs. The values here may not be 100% accurate because the recipes have not been professionally evaluated nor have they been evaluated by the U.S. FDA.

Cheeseburger Soup

Serves 6

Prep and cook time: 55 minutes

Ingredients:

- 1 1/2 lbs. ground bison or ground grass fed beef
- 3 tbsp. avocado oil
- 1 medium yellow onion, diced
- 1 cup green beans, diced
- 1 16 oz. can diced tomatoes in juice
- 5 cups water or vegetable broth

- 1 tbsp. Cumin
- 1 tsp. Onion powder
- 2 cloves garlic, diced
- 1/2 cup shredded organic cheddar, cream cheese or cheese of choice

Directions:

1. In large stock pot add oil, onion, garlic and seasonings. Cook over low heat while stirring for 5 minutes.
2. Add in ground bison. Stir while cooking on medium until all meat is browned.
3. Add remaining ingredients and cover. Simmer for 35 minutes.
4. Stir in cheese and cook for 5 minutes on low while stirring.
5. Serve in bowls.

Nutrition Facts

Servings 6.0

Amount Per Serving calories 474

% Daily Value *

Total Fat 37 g   56 %

Saturated Fat 16 g   80 %

Monounsaturated Fat 8 g

Polyunsaturated Fat 1 g

Trans Fat 0 g

Cholesterol 115 mg   38 %

Sodium 880 mg	37 %
Potassium 186 mg	5 %
Total Carbohydrate 6 g	2 %
Dietary Fiber 1 g	4 %
Sugars 1 g	
Protein 30 g	61 %
Vitamin A	16 %
Vitamin C	7 %
Calcium	37 %
Iron	21 %

*   The Percent Daily Values are based on a 2,000 calorie diet, so your values may change depending on your calorie needs. The values here may not be 100% accurate because the recipes have not been professionally evaluated nor have they been evaluated by the U.S. FDA.

Cream of Mushroom Soup

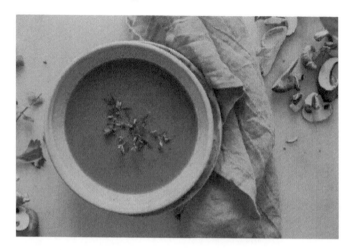

Serves 6

Prep and cook time: 35 minutes

Ingredients:

- 2 lbs. Mixed mushrooms (button, cremini, shitake, portabella)
- 2 tbsp. butter
- 4 cups vegetable broth
- 2 cloves garlic diced
- 3 shallots, peeled, diced finely
- 1/2 cup heavy whipping cream
- 1 tsp. Onion powder
- 1 tsp. Fresh tarragon, chopped
- Sea salt and pepper to taste

Directions

1. In a large stock pot, melt butter and add garlic, shallots, and seasonings except for tarragon.

2.   Saute for 5 minutes on medium heat.
3.   Add mushrooms and saute for 5 minutes, while stirring.
4.   Add in broth and cover. Reduce heat to low and simmer for 20 minutes.
5.   Add in whipping cream and stir.
6.   Add tarragon, and simmer on low for an additional 5 minutes.
7.   Serve immediately.

Nutrition Facts

Servings 6.0

Amount Per Serving calories 170

% Daily Value *

Total Fat 15 g	24 %
Saturated Fat 7 g	35 %
Monounsaturated Fat 3 g	
Polyunsaturated Fat 0 g	
Trans Fat 0 g	
Cholesterol 38 mg	13 %
Sodium 939 mg	39 %
Potassium 57 mg	2 %
Total Carbohydrate 9 g	3 %
Dietary Fiber 1 g	4 %
Sugars 3 g	

Protein 1 g	3 %
Vitamin A	38 %
Vitamin C	5 %
Calcium	5 %
Iron	1 %

*   The Percent Daily Values are based on a 2,000 calorie diet, so your values may change depending on your calorie needs. The values here may not be 100% accurate because the recipes have not been professionally evaluated nor have they been evaluated by the U.S. FDA

Classic Chicken Egg Drop Soup

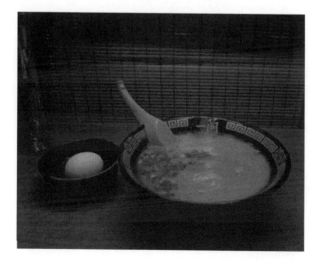

Serves 4

Cook time: 40 minutes

Ingredients:

- 2 chicken breast fillets, cut into small pieces
- 4 cups chicken broth
- 1 tsp. Avocado oil
- 2 eggs
- 1 " piece of ginger, peeled and finely diced
- 2 scallions, chopped
- 1 carrot, peeled and sliced thinly
- 1 clove garlic, finely diced
- 1 cup cabbage, shredded
- 1/2 tsp. Salt
- Pepper to taste

Directions:

1. In a large stock pot, heat oil, ginger, scallions, garlic, cabbage, and carrots.
2. Simmer on low for 5 minutes.
3. Add remaining ingredients, except for eggs.
4. Cover and simmer on low for 25 minutes.
5. Meanwhile, beat eggs in a bowl.
6. Uncover soup, and bring to a low boil.
7. Slowly drop egg mixture into soup by spoonfuls, while stirring.
8. Cook for 5 more minutes.
9. Serve immediately.

Nutrition Facts

Servings 4.0

Amount Per Serving calories 179

% Daily Value *

Total Fat 5 g	7 %
Saturated Fat 1 g	6 %
Monounsaturated Fat 2 g	
Polyunsaturated Fat 1 g	
Trans Fat 0 g	
Cholesterol 125 mg	42 %
Sodium 403 mg	17 %
Potassium 193 mg	6 %
Total Carbohydrate 10 g	3 %
Dietary Fiber 2 g	9 %
Sugars 3 g	
Protein 17 g	35 %
Vitamin A	60 %
Vitamin C	22 %
Calcium	15 %
Iron	6 %

*   The Percent Daily Values are based on a 2,000 calorie diet, so your values may change depending on your calorie needs. The values here may not be 100% accurate because the recipes have not been professionally evaluated nor have they been evaluated by the U.S. FDA.

Italian Bacon and Vegetable Soup

Serves 6

Prep and cook time: 55 minutes

Ingredients:

- 6 Cups organic vegetable broth
- 4 slices bacon, cut into pieces
- 1 cup green beans, cut in half
- 1 Medium yellow onion, diced
- 1 8 oz. can diced tomatoes in juice
- 2 Carrots sliced
- 2 yellow zucchini diced
- 1 red pepper, seeded, sliced thin
- 1 cup spinach, packed
- 3 cloves garlic, chopped
- 1 tbsp. Oregano
- 2 tsp. Basil
- 1 bay leaf
- 2 Tbsp. sea salt
- 1/2 tsp. Fresh ground pepper
- 3 Tbsp. Avocado Oil
- 1/2 tsp. Red pepper flakes (optional)
- 2 tbsp. Fresh Italian Parsley (for garnish)

Directions:

1.   In large stockpot, heat oil and bacon, garlic, onion, vegetables and seasonings on low for 5 minutes.
2.   Add in remainder of ingredients, except for the broth.
3.   Bring to a low boil for an additional 5 minutes.
4.   Add broth and cover. Simmer for 40 minutes on low, or until vegetables are tender. Remove bay leaf. Add red pepper flakes if using.
5.   Serve in bowls, garnish with parsley.

Nutrition Facts

Servings 6.0

Amount Per Serving calories 138

% Daily Value *

Total Fat 10 g   15 %

Saturated Fat 2 g   9 %

Monounsaturated Fat 6 g

Polyunsaturated Fat 2 g

Trans Fat 0 g

Cholesterol 5 mg   2 %

Sodium 2674 mg   111 %

Potassium 374 mg   11 %

Total Carbohydrate 10 g   3 %

Dietary Fiber 3g   11%

Sugars 5 g

Protein 3 g 7%

Vitamin A 119 %

Vitamin C 65 %

Calcium 17 %

Iron 8 %

*   The Percent Daily Values are based on a 2,000 calorie diet, so your values may change depending on your calorie needs. The values here may not be 100% accurate because the recipes have not been professionally evaluated nor have they been evaluated by the U.S. FDA.

Cream of Broccoli Soup

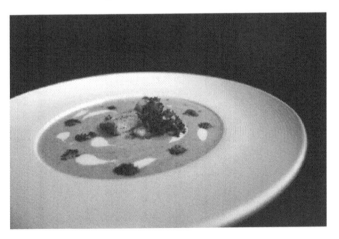

Serves 6

Cook time: 40 minutes

Ingredients

- 3 tbsp. butter
- 1 small yellow onion, diced
- 2 celery stalks, chopped
- 3 cups broccoli florets
- 3 cups vegetable broth
- 1 cup full fat sour cream or 1 cup unsweetened coconut milk
- 1 tsp. Sea salt
- Pepper to taste

Directions

1. Heat the butter in a large pot and sauté onion, broccoli and celery for about 4-5 minutes.
2. Add in broth, and salt. Cover and simmer for 20 minutes.
3. Add sour cream (or coconut milk) and simmer for an additional 5 minutes, while stirring.
4. Turn off heat, and either use a submersion blender to blend all ingredients until creamy. Or, slowly take by the cupful and add to a blender...(watch out, it will be hot!)
5. and blend for 30 seconds then transfer back to the pot.
6. Serve immediately.
7.

Nutrition Facts

Servings 6.0

Amount Per Serving calories 128

% Daily Value *

Total Fat 11 g   17 %

Saturated Fat 7 g   35 %

Monounsaturated Fat 2 g

Polyunsaturated Fat 0 g

Trans Fat 0 g

Cholesterol 35 mg	12 %
Sodium 392 mg	16 %
Potassium 72 mg	2%
Total Carbohydrate 4g	1%
Dietary Fiber 1 g	3%

Sugars 2 g

Protein 1 g	3 %
Vitamin A	53 %
Vitamin C	19 %
Calcium	5%
Iron	2 %

*   The Percent Daily Values are based on a 2,000 calorie diet, so your values may change depending on your calorie needs. The values here may not be 100% accurate because the recipes have not been professionally evaluated nor have they been evaluated by the U.S. FDA.

Cream of Pumpkin Spice Soup (crock-pot)

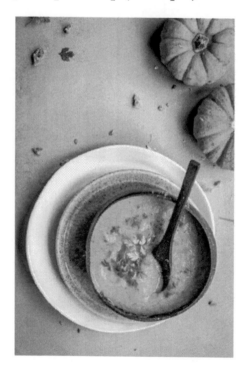

Serves 8

Prep and Cook time: 8 hours

Ingredients

- 4 lbs. Pumpkin, peeled and diced into large chunks
- 4 cups organic vegetable stock or broth
- 1 Cup flax or unsweetened almond milk
- 1 cup full-fat cream (save this for the last step)
- 4 Tbsp. grass fed butter
- 1 clove garlic
- 1 small yellow onion diced
- 1 Tbsp. Sea salt
- 1 tsp. nutmeg
- 1 tsp. paprika
- 1 tsp. fresh ground pepper

Directions

1. Add all ingredients into slow cooker. Cover and cook on low for 6-8 hours.
2. Pour in cream and coconut milk and blend by hand.
3. Use immersion handheld blender in the slow cooker to puree all ingredients. Or, you can pour the mixture carefully in small batches (it's hot!) into a blender to puree and blend all ingredients.

Nutrition Facts

Servings 8.0

Amount Per Serving calories 165

% Daily Value *

Total Fat 11 g   18 %

Saturated Fat 8 g   38 %

Monounsaturated Fat 0 g

Polyunsaturated Fat 0 g

Trans Fat 0 g

Cholesterol 35 mg	12 %
Sodium 1388 mg	58 %
Potassium 434 mg	12 %
Total Carbohydrate 12 g	4 %
Dietary Fiber 1g	4%
Sugars 6 g	
Protein 2 g	5 %
Vitamin A	214 %
Vitamin C	18 %
Calcium	10 %
Iron	6 %

*   The Percent Daily Values are based on a 2,000 calorie diet, so your values may change depending on your calorie needs. The values here may not be 100% accurate because the recipes have not been professionally evaluated nor have they been evaluated by the U.S. FDA.

Creamy Coconut Curry Chicken Soup

Serves 4

Cook and Prep time: 45 minutes.

Ingredients

- 2 Chicken breasts, cut into chunks
- 3 Tbsp. Coconut Oil
- 1 cup vegetable broth
- 1 cups flax or unsweetened almond milk
- 1 - 13.5 oz cans full fat coconut milk
- 2 Tsp. salt
- 3⁄4 Tsp red pepper flakes
- 2 tbsp. curry
- 1 tsp. cumin
- 1 Large yellow onion, chopped
- 8 Cloves garlic minced
- 1/4 Cup fresh cilantro, chopped
- 1 tsp. Sea salt
- Pepper to taste

Directions:

1. Saute chicken, onions, garlic, seasonings, and salt in coconut oil for 10 minutes on low.
2. Add broth and flax milk, and cover. Simmer for 30 minutes.
3. Add coconut milk and stir to blend.
4. Simmer for an additional 10 minutes.
5. Add salt and pepper and top with fresh cilantro before serving.

Nutrition Facts

Servings 4.0

Amount Per Serving calories 278

% Daily Value *

Total Fat 18 g	28 %
Saturated Fat 13 g	64 %
Monounsaturated Fat 2 g	
Polyunsaturated Fat 1 g	
Trans Fat 0 g	
Cholesterol 49 mg	16 %
Sodium 2086 mg	87 %
Potassium 362 mg	10 %
Total Carbohydrate 8 g	3 %
Dietary Fiber 2 g	10 %
Sugars 5 g	
Protein 21 g	43 %
Vitamin A	11 %
Vitamin C	2 %
Calcium	21 %
Iron	10 %

*   The Percent Daily Values are based on a 2,000 calorie diet, so your values may change depending on your calorie needs. The values here may not be 100% accurate because the recipes have not been professionally evaluated nor have they been evaluated by the U.S. FDA.

Gazpacho

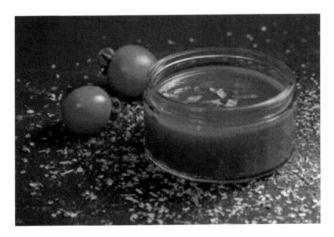

Serves 6

Prep time: 20 minutes

Ingredients:

- 5 cups vine ripened tomatoes, diced
- 2 long, seedless cucumbers, peeled and diced
- 1/4 cup red onion, diced
- 1 garlic clove, chopped
- 1/2 cup. Avocado oil
- 1/3 cup. Vinegar
- 1 tsp. Spanish paprika
- 1 bunch cilantro, chopped, stems removed

- 1/4 tsp. Worcestershire sauce
- Salt and pepper to taste

Directions:

1. Blend all ingredients together by pulsing on low, 3-4 times in a food processor, except for avocado oil, salt and pepper.
2. Add oil, pulse until desired consistency.
3. Add salt and pepper to taste.

Nutrition Facts

Servings 6.0

Amount Per Serving calories 145

% Daily Value *

Total Fat 12 g	18 %
Saturated Fat 2 g	9 %
Monounsaturated Fat 8 g	
Polyunsaturated Fat 2 g	
Trans Fat 0 g	
Cholesterol 0 mg	0 %
Sodium 60 mg	3 %
Potassium 377 mg	11%

Total Carbohydrate7 g   2 %

Dietary Fiber 2 g   7%

Sugars 4 g

Protein 1 g   2 %

Vitamin A   62 %

Vitamin C   18 %

Calcium   16%

Iron   1 %

*   The Percent Daily Values are based on a 2,000 calorie diet, so your values may change depending on your calorie needs. The values here may not be 100% accurate because the recipes have not been professionally evaluated nor have they been evaluated by the U.S. FDA.

Healing Garden Vegetable Soup

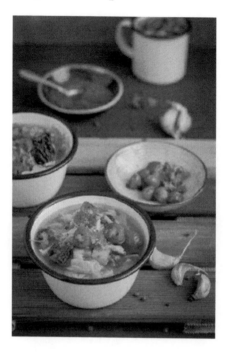

Serves 6

Cook and Prep time: 1 hour 15 minutes

Ingredients:

- 6 cups vegetable broth
- 3 tbsp. Olive oil
- 3 cloves garlic, sliced thin
- 2 yellow squash, cut into cubes
- 1 large yellow onion, diced
- 8 cherry tomatoes, cut into halves
- 1 baby eggplant, cut into cubes
- 1 cup mixed mushrooms

- 2 cups spinach
- 1 tbsp. Cayenne pepper
- 1 tsp. Cumin
- 1 tsp. Turmeric powder
- 1 tsp. Sea salt
- Salt and pepper to taste

Directions:

1. In a large stock pot, heat oil, garlic, tomatoes, onion, spinach and mushrooms. Stir for 10 minutes.
2. Add in salt, seasonings, and eggplant.
3. Cook while stirring for an additional 5 minutes.
4. Add remainder of ingredients, including broth.
5. Cover and simmer for 40 minutes.
6. Serve immediately in bowls.

Nutrition Facts

Servings 6.0

Amount Per Serving calories 121

% Daily Value *

Total Fat 8 g   13 %

Saturated Fat 1 g   6 %

Monounsaturated Fat 6 g

Polyunsaturated Fat 1 g

Trans Fat 0 g

Cholesterol 0 mg	0 %
Sodium 1401 mg	58 %
Potassium 490 mg	14%
Total Carbohydrate 10 g	3 %
Dietary Fiber 2 g	7%
Sugars 7 g	
Protein 3 g	5 %
Vitamin A	86 %
Vitamin C	42 %
Calcium	15%
Iron	5 %

*   The Percent Daily Values are based on a 2,000 calorie diet, so your values may change depending on your calorie needs. The values here may not be 100% accurate because the recipes have not been professionally evaluated nor have they been evaluated by the U.S. FDA.

Lobster Bisque

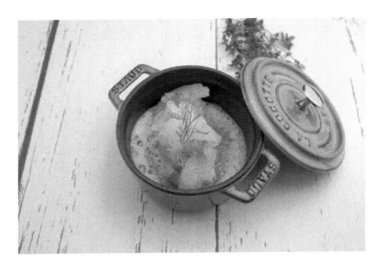

Serves 6

Prep and Cook time: 40 minutes

Ingredients:

- 1 lb. cooked lobster meat, chopped
- 4 tbsp. butter
- 1 cup unsweetened flax milk
- 1 cups vegetable broth
- 2 tbsp. dry white cooking wine, or Sherry
- 1 carrot peeled, sliced thin
- 3 stalks celery, diced
- 1 clove garlic, diced
- 1 cup heavy whipping cream
- 1 tsp. Celery salt
- 1 tsp. Dried thyme
- Salt and pepper to taste

Directions:

1.   In a large stock pot, melt butter, and add in, garlic, celery, carrots and seasonings. Cook on low for 5 minutes.

2.   Add a 1/2 cup of the broth, the lobster, and cook on low, covered for 5 minutes.

3.   Add milk and wine. Cover and cook for 15 minutes. Stirring occasionally.

4.   Add cream and continue to simmer for an additional 15 minutes.

5.   Add salt and pepper to taste after serving in bowls.

Nutrition Facts

Servings 6.0

Amount Per Serving calories 226

% Daily Value *

Total Fat 18 g	28 %
Saturated Fat 12 g	59 %
Monounsaturated Fat 2 g	
Polyunsaturated Fat 1 g	
Trans Fat 0 g	
Cholesterol 60 mg	20 %
Sodium 713 mg	30 %
Potassium 6 mg	0%
Total Carbohydrate 6 g	2 %
Dietary Fiber 0 g	2%
Sugars 1 g	

Protein 9 g	18 %
Vitamin A	114 %
Vitamin C	1 %
Calcium	12%
Iron	7 %

* The Percent Daily Values are based on a 2,000 calorie diet, so your values may change depending on your calorie needs. The values here may not be 100% accurate because the recipes have not been professionally evaluated nor have they been evaluated by the U.S. FDA.

20 KETO SMOOTHIE RECIPES

1.   **Peanut Butter Coconut Smoothie**

Ingredients:

*   ½ cup coconut milk, unsweetened, canned

*   ¼ avocado, frozen

*   ½ tbsp peanut butter

*   ½ tbsp chia seeds, soaked

*   1 tsp cocoa powder, unsweetened

*   ½ tbsp coconut oil

*   ice/water if needed

*   ½ tbsp coconut flakes for decoration

Nutritional Information and Health Benefits:

Energy: 464.5 kcal, Protein: 6.8 g, Fat: 4.7 g, Net Carbs: 6.1 g

This smoothie is rich in omega-3 fatty acids, antioxidants, fiber, iron and calcium. It is also an excellent source of vitamin B2, B3, B5 and B6. The drink is a source of manganese, phosphorus, copper, selenium as well as magnesium.

2.   Carrot Smoothie

Ingredients:

- ¼ cup coconut milk, unsweetened, canned

- ½ a medium carrot

- ¼ cup coconut yogurt, unsweetened

- 1 tbsp sesame seed tahini

- ½ tsp stevia or another low-carb sweetener

- ¼ tsp cinnamon, ground

- 1/8 tsp nutmeg

- ice (optional)

Nutritional Information and Health Benefits:

Energy: 241.5 kcal, Protein: 14.5 g, Fat: 21.9 g, Net Carbs: 6.8 g

This smoothie is rich in beta-carotene, easily convertible to vitamin A in the body. Furthermore, it is an excellent source of vitamin K, potassium, vitamin E and vitamin B6. This drink is rich in antioxidants, has anti-inflammatory and antibacterial properties, strengthens the immune system, protects the liver and kidney function.

3.   Protein Strawberry Smoothie

Ingredients:

- 1/2 cup coconut milk, unsweetened, canned

- ½ cup strawberries, frozen

- ½ scoop protein powder (of any choice, preferably strawberry flavor or vanilla, chocolate is also possible)

- 1 tbsp coconut oil

- ¼ tsp stevia or another low-carb sweetener

- 1 tbsp lime juice

Nutritional Information and Health Benefits:

Energy: 426 kcal, Protein: 35.5 g, Fat: 36.8 g, Net Carbs: 10 g

This smoothie is rich protein, vitamin C, manganese, folate, potassium and antioxidants. It also has some amounts of iron, calcium and vitamin B6.

4.   Fresh Cucumber Smoothie

Ingredients:

- 1 cucumber (around 200 g)

- ½ avocado

- a pinch of sea salt

- juice of ½ lemon

- ½ parsley sprig

- water as much as you want

Nutritional Information and Health Benefits:

Energy: 196 kcal, Protein: 3.6 g, Fat: 15.3 g, Net Carbs: 9.8 g

This smoothie is rich in dietary fiber, folate, iron, magnesium, potassium, vitamin C as well as vitamin B2, B3 and B5.

5. Detox Smoothie with Spirulina

Ingredients:

- ½ cucumber (around 100 g)

- ¼ cup spinach

- 1 slice of celery head

- juice of ½ lemon

- one 5 mm slice ginger

- ½ avocado

- 1 tsp wheat grass

- 1 tsp spirulina

Nutritional Information and Health Benefits:

Energy: 199.4 kcal, Protein: 6.1 g, Fat: 15.2 g, Net Carbs: 8.6 g

This smoothie is an excellent source of vitamin K, vitamin A, vitamin C, iron, magnesium, vitamin B2, B3, B5. It is also very rich in fiber and potassium.

6. Blueberry Chocolate Protein Smoothie

Ingredients:

- 1 cup almond milk, unsweetened
- ¼ cup blueberries
- 1 tsp vanilla extract
- 1 tsp coconut oil
- ½ scoop protein powder, chocolate flavor

Nutritional Information and Health Benefits:

Energy: 216 kcal, Protein: 25 g, Fat: 7.2 g, Net Carbs: 7 g

This smoothie is rich in protein, copper, beta-carotene, folate, choline, vitamins A and E, as well as manganese. It also prevents tooth decay, due to the properties of vanilla.

7. Green Tea Smoothie

Ingredients:

- ½ cup green tea, chilled
- ½ cup spinach leaves
- ½ kiwi, peeled

- 1/8 avocado

- ¼ small banana

- ¼ tsp ginger, ground

Nutritional Information and Health Benefits:

Energy: 86.5 kcal, Protein: 1.7 g, Fat: 4.1 g, Net Carbs: 10 g

This smoothie is a healthy source of fiber, potassium, vitamin B6, B5, B3 and B2, vitamin C, vitamin K, vitamin E, folate, as well as antioxidants, iron and magnesium. This healthy drink reduces muscle soreness and pain and has anti-inflammatory effects.

8.   Berry Smoothie

Ingredients:

- 1 cup berry mix, frozen

- ½ cup almond milk, unsweetened

- 1 tbsp chia seeds, soaked

- ½ cup ice cubes, crushed

Nutritional Information and Health Benefits:

Energy: 151 kcal, Protein: 3.9 g, Fat: 4 g, Net Carbs: 9.9 g

This smoothie is rich in omega-3 fatty acids, antioxidants, fiber, iron and calcium. It is also a great source of manganese, phosphorus, copper, selenium and magnesium.

9. Raspberry Cheesecake Smoothie

Ingredients:

- 2 tbsp cream cheese, softened

- ½ cup almond milk, unsweetened

- ¼ cup whipped cream

- ¾ cup raspberries, frozen

- 1 rich tea biscuit (Maria Cookie for example)

- ½ cup ice cubes, crushed

Nutritional Information and Health Benefits:

Energy: 388.8 kcal, Protein: 5.4 g, Fat: 33.4 g, Net Carbs: 11.9 g

This smoothie is very rich in antioxidants, as well as vitamin C and vitamin K. It also has some vitamin E, manganese and vitamin B6.

10. Tomato Detox Smoothie

Ingredients:

- 1 ½ cup spinach

- 1 tomato small

- 1 carrot

- ½ beet beetroot

- ½ stalk celery

- 1 sprig parsley

- water

Nutritional Information and Health Benefits:

Energy: 67.5 kcal, Protein: 3.7 g, Fat: 0.5 g, Net Carbs: 9.6 g

This smoothie an excellent source of vitamin K, vitamin A, vitamin C, iron, magnesium, vitamin B2, potassium, fiber, folate and beta-carotene.

11. Vanilla Strawberry Smoothie

Ingredients:

- 1 cup coconut milk, unsweetened, canned

- juice from ½ lemon

- ½ tsp vanilla extract

- 5 strawberries

- ice (optional)

Nutritional Information and Health Benefits:

Energy: 426 kcal, Protein: 5 g, Fat: 48.3 g, Net Carbs: 10 g

This smoothie is very rich in antioxidants, vitamin C, manganese, folate and potassium. It helps prevention of tooth decay.

12.   Blueberry Spinach Smoothie

Ingredients:

*   1/3 cup blueberries

*   ½ cup spinach

*   ¼ small banana

*   1 cup almond milk, unsweetened

Nutritional Information and Health Benefits:

Energy: 84 kcal, Protein: 2.2 g, Fat: 2.9 g, Net Carbs: 11 g

This low-calorie smoothie is a great source of fiber, potassium, vitamin B6, vitamin C, vitamin A, vitamin K, iron, magnesium, vitamin B2 and manganese. It is also rich in copper, beta-carotene and folate.

13.   Fresh Kiwi and Lettuce Smoothie

Ingredients:

*   ¾ kiwi, peeled

*   ¼ bulb fennel

*   ¼ avocado

*   1/3 cup lettuce

*   ½ cup water (and/or some ice)

Nutritional Information and Health Benefits:

Energy: 131.5 kcal, Protein: 2.5 g, Fat: 7.9 g, Net Carbs: 9.7 g

This smoothie is a great source of fiber, vitamin C, vitamin K, vitamin E, vitamin A, folate, as well as antioxidants, magnesium, potassium, selenium, copper, zinc and vitamins B2, B3, B5 and B6.

14. Seed Smoothie with Greens

Ingredients:

- ½ cup almond milk, unsweetened

- ½ cup kale

- 1 ½ cup spinach

- ¼ small banana

- 3 strawberries

- ½ tbsp chia seeds, soaked (preferably)

- 1 tsp hemp seeds

- ice

Nutritional Information and Health Benefits:

Energy: 113.5 kcal, Protein: 5.2 g, Fat: 5.8 g, Net Carbs: 10.4 g

This smoothie is an excellent source of source of fiber, potassium, vitamin B6, vitamin C, vitamin A. The chia seeds provide iron and calcium and are full of omega-3 fatty acids, as well as folate. It has also vitamin K, essential for maintaining bone health. The smoothie also contains copper, selenium and phosphorus. This drink is also a source of healthy fats and zinc.

15.   Fantastic Yellow Spiced Smoothie

Ingredients:

- 1/2 cup coconut milk, unsweetened, canned

- 1 cup almond milk, unsweetened

- 1 tsp stevia or another low-carb sweetener

- 1 tbsp turmeric, ground

- 1 tsp ginger, ground

- 1 tsp cinnamon, ground

- 1 tbsp coconut oil

- 1 tbsp chia seeds, soaked

Nutritional Information and Health Benefits:

Energy: 481 kcal, Protein: 6.5 g, Fat: 45.6 g, Net Carbs: 8.4 g

This smoothie is an excellent course of omega-3 fatty acids, fiber, iron and calcium. It is also rich in antioxidants, manganese, phosphorus, copper, selenium and magnesium. It has anti-inflammatory properties and reduces muscle soreness and pain.

16. Green Low Calorie Smoothie

Ingredients:

- 2 thin slices pineapple

- juice from ¼ lemon

- 6 spinach leaves

- ½ cup water

- ¼ tsp ginger, ground

Nutritional Information and Health Benefits:

Energy: 46 kcal, Protein: 6 g, Fat: 0.2 g, Net Carbs: 9.9 g

This smoothie is an excellent source of vitamin K, vitamin A, vitamin C, iron, magnesium, vitamin B2 and potassium. This healthy drink possesses anti-inflammatory properties and cures muscle soreness and pain.

17. Cocoa Coconut Smoothie with Blackberries

Ingredients:

- 1 cup coconut milk, unsweetened, canned

- ½ tsp stevia or another low-carb sweetener

- 1/8 avocado

- ¼ cup blackberries

- ½ tsp chia seeds, soaked

- 1 tsp cocoa powder, unsweetened

- ½ tbsp almond butter

Nutritional Information and Health Benefits:

Energy: 565.5 kcal, Protein: 7.9 g, Fat: 57.5 g, Net Carbs: 9.2 g

This smoothie is rich in omega-3 fatty acids, antioxidants, fiber, iron and calcium, vitamin B2, B3 and B5. It is also a source of vitamin A and C, as well as manganese, potassium, phosphorus, copper, selenium and magnesium.

18.   Raspberry Pure Coconut Smoothie

Ingredients:

- 1 cup almond milk, unsweetened

- 1 cup raspberries

- 1 tbsp chia seeds, soaked

- ¼ tsp cinnamon, ground

- 1 tsp coconut flakes

Nutritional Information and Health Benefits:

Energy: 208.5 kcal, Protein: 4.9 g, Fat: 11.9 g, Net Carbs: 8.5 g

This smoothie is a great source of omega-3 fatty acids, antioxidants, fiber, iron and calcium. It is also very rich in vitamin C and vitamin K. The drink has some vitamin E, manganese and vitamin B6, selenium, copper and phosphorus.

19.   Chocolate Smoothie with Greens

Ingredients:

• ½ cup coconut milk, unsweetened, canned

• 1 slice zucchini

• ¼ cup spinach

• ¼ cup romaine lettuce

• ½ avocado

• 1 tbsp chia seeds, soaked

• 2 tbsp cocoa powder

Nutritional Information and Health Benefits:

Energy: 489 kcal, Protein: 8.7 g, Fat: 44.8 g, Net Carbs: 8.4 g

This smoothie is rich in vitamin C, vitamin K, folic acid, iron and calcium. It is also a source of vitamin B2, B5, B3, magnesium, potassium, fiber, copper, phosphorous and selenium. This smoothie improves the nitric oxide levels, improves blood flow and brain function and may improve symptoms of type 2 diabetes, due to the benefits of cocoa.

20. Super Low Carb Green Tahini Smoothie

Ingredients:

- ¼ cup spinach

- ¼ cup arugula

- juice of ½ lemon

- 1 tbsp sesame tahini

- 3 stalks celery

- water according to preference

- stevia or another artificial sweetener (optional)

Nutritional Information and Health Benefits:

Energy: 97.3 kcal, Protein: 3.6 g, Fat: 8.4 g, Net Carbs: 2.8 g

This smoothie is an excellent source of vitamin C, vitamin K, vitamin A, potassium, phosphorus, manganese, folic acid, iron and calcium. The drink has antibacterial properties, has anti-inflammatory compounds and strengthens the central nervous system. Furthermore, it also protects the liver and kidney function and may have anticancer effects.

IMMUNITY BOOSTING SOUPS

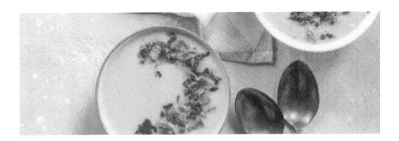

Crispy Prosciutto & Leek Soup

4 serving 30 minutes

Ingredients

- ½ tsp Avocado Oil
- 2 Leeks (trimmed, roughly chopped)
- ½ Yellow Onion (chopped)
- ½ head Cauliflower (cut into florets)
- 4 cups Organic Chicken Broth
- ½ tsp Sea Salt
- 4 ozs Prosciutto (sliced into small pieces)
- 1 ¼ cups Organic Coconut Milk (full fat, canned)
- ¼ Parsley (chopped)

Directions

1. In a large pot or dutch oven, heat the avocado oil over medium heat. Once hot, add the leeks and onion and sauté for 4 to 5 minutes. Add the cauliflower, chicken broth and sea salt. Bring to a boil, then reduce heat and let simmer for 15 to 18 minutes.

2. Meanwhile, heat a large non-stick skillet over medium heat. Add the prosciutto and cook for 3 minutes per side or until crisp. Remove from the pan and set aside.

3. Add the coconut milk to the soup and stir to incorporate. Blend the soup with a stick blender or in a blender. Ladle into bowls and top with crispy prosciutto and parsley. Serve and enjoy!

Nutrtion

- Amount per serving
- Calories 266g
- Fat 18g
- Carbs 15g
- Fiber 3g
- Sugar 6g
- Protein 12g
- Sodium 1796mg

Notes

Leftovers, Refrigerate in an airtight container for up to three days. Freeze for up to three months.

Serving Size, One serving is equal to approximately 1.5 cups of soup.

More Flavor, Add black pepper or your favorite herbs and spices to the soup. Omit, or use crispy bacon instead.

Make it vegan, Use vegetable broth and omit the prosciutto.

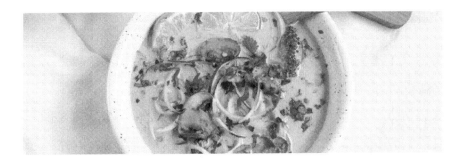

Curried Coconut Soup

8 Serving 30 minutes

Ingredients

- 1 ½ tsps. Coconut Oil
- 1 Garlic (clove, minced)
- 1tsp Ginger (minced)
- 3 cups Organic Chicken Broth
- ¼ oz Lemongrass (peeled, chopped into large pieces)
- 8 ozs Chicken Breast (skinless, boneless, chopped into cubes)
- 1 ½ cups Shiitake Mushrooms (sliced)
- 1 cup Organic Coconut Milk (canned)
- 1tbsp Lime Juice
- ¼ cup Thai Basli (chopped)

Nutrition

Amount per serving

- Calories 478g
- Fat 29g

124

- Carbs 24g
- Fiber   2g
- Sugar 9g
- Protein 31g
- Sodium1607mg

Directions

1. In a pot over medium heat, add the coconut oil, garlic and ginger. Sauté for 1 minute. Then add the broth, coconut aminos and lemongrass. Bring to a simmer, reduce heat to medium-low and cook for 15 to 20 minutes

2. Add the chicken and mushrooms and cook for 10 minutes or until the chicken is cooked through. Remove from heat. Remove the lemongrass stalks and discard. Add the coconut milk and lime juice. Stir to combine.

3. Divide into bowls and garnish with basil. Enjoy!

Notes

Leftovers, Refrigerate in an airtight container for up to five days.

Additional Toppings, Add leafy greens such as spinach or kale.

No Lemongrass, Use extra lime juice instead.

No Coconut Aminos, Use tamari or soy sauce instead.

No Thai Basil, Use regular basil, cilantro or mint instead.

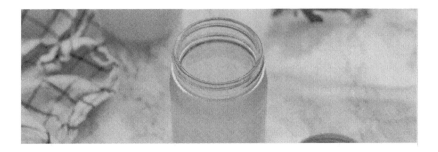

Pressure Cooker Bone Broth

4 serving 3 hours

Ingredients

- 1 Whole Chicken Carcass
- 2 Carrot (medium, chopped)
- 1 Yellow Onion (chopped)
- 1 tbsp Apple Cider Vinegar
- 1 tsp Sea Salt
- 5 cups Water

Nutrition

- Amount per serving
- Calories 25g
- Fat 0g
- Carbs 6g
- Fiber   2g
- Sugar 4g
- Protein 1g
- Sodium618mg

Directions

1. Add the cooked chicken carcass/bones to the pressure cooker along with the carrots, onion, apple cider vinegar and sea salt.

2. Add the water to the pressure cooker. Lock the lid on and make

sure the knob is set to the "sealing" position. Select the "manual" or "pressure cook" (on newer models) setting and set for two hours.

3. Once the two hours are up, allow the pressure to release naturally. Then open the lid carefully and strain the broth through a sieve or strainer. Discard the veggies and bones then transfer the broth into jars. Enjoy!

Notes

Chicken Carcass, One whole chicken carcass is equal to about 2 lbs. of bones.

Layer of Fat, A layer of fat may form on the top of the broth once it cools. You can keep it or skim it off once it has hardened.

Storage, Store broth in the fridge for up to 3 to 4 days or freeze until ready to use. For easy freezing, pour into an ice cube tray and freeze, then remove and place in a bag in the freezer.

No Onion, Omit or use celery for extra flavour instead.

Save Your Bones, Anytime you have extra bones from a meal, freeze them for when you are ready to make broth.

Use it With, You can use this broth in soups, stews, curries, quinoa or simply sip it on its own.

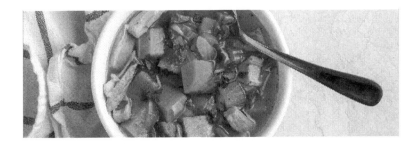

Turkey & Vegetable Soup

6 serving 50 minutes

Ingredients

- 1 tbsp Extra Virgin Olive Oil
- 1 Yellow Onion (chopped)
- 3 Garlic (clove, minced)
- 1tsp Dried Thyme
- 1 tsp Sea Salt
- 1 Sweet Potato (peeled, cut into 1/2- inch cubes)
- 1Carrot (peeled, chopped)
- 2 stalks Celery (chopped)
- 10 ½ ozs Turkey Breast, Cooked (roughly chopped)
- 6 cups Organic Chicken Broth
- 1 cup Parsley (chopped)

Nutrition

- Amount per serving
- Calories 142g
- Fat 4g
- Carbs 10g
- Fiber   2g
- Sugar 4g
- Protein 18g
- Sodium1411mg

Directions

1. Heat the oil in a large pot over medium heat.

2. Add the onion and cook until it begins to soften, about 5 minutes. Add in the garlic, thyme and salt and continue cooking for one minute more.

3. Add the sweet potato, carrots, celery and turkey. Stir to combine then add the chicken broth to the pot along with the parsley.

4. Bring soup to a gentle boil then reduce the heat to low and cover with a lid. Simmer for 40 to 45 minutes or until the vegetables are very tender. Season with additional salt if needed. Serve and enjoy!

Notes

Leftovers, Refrigerate in an airtight container for up to three days.

Serving Size, One serving is approximately 1 1/2 cups of soup.

More Flavor, Add a bay leaf or some red pepper flakes.

No Turkey, Use chicken breast instead.

Additional Toppings, Serve the soup over top of cooked rice or cooked pasta.

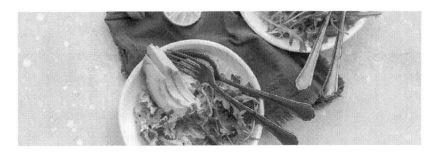

Ingredients

- 1Ib Chicken Thighs (boneless, skinless)
- 1/3 tsp Dried Thyme
- ½ tsp Onion Powder
- ½ Sea Salt (divided)
- 2 tsps Avocado Oil (divided)
- ½ Yellow Onion (chopped)
- 2 stalks Celery (chopped)
- 2 Garlic (cloves, minced)
- 1 ¼ cups Organic Chicken Broth
- 1 ¼ cups Organic Coconut Milk (full fat, from a can)
- 2 tbsps Lime Juice Arugula
- 1 Avocado (sliced)

Nutrition

- Amount per serving
- Calories 392g
- Fat 28g
- Carbs 10g
- Fiber   4g
- Sugar 3g
- Protein 25g
- Sodium734mg

Directions

1. In a shallow dish, add the chicken breast and season with thyme,

onion powder, half the sea salt and half the avocado oil.

2. In a dutch oven, over medium heat, add the remaining avocado oil along with the onion and celery and cook for 5 minutes. Add the garlic and cook for 1 minute more. Add the chicken to the pot and brown on all sides, about 5 to 7 minutes.

3. Add the broth and lower the heat to medium-low and let it simmer for about 10 minutes. Remove the chicken and shred it using two forks. Return to the pot along with the coconut milk, lime juice and remaining sea salt and stir to combine.

4. Divide the chicken into bowls and top with arugula and avocado. Enjoy!

Notes

Leftovers, Refrigerate in an airtight container for up to three days.

More Flavor, Add mushroom powder to season the chicken. Top with chili flakes for more spice.

Additional Toppings, Serve with tortilla chips for dipping.

Creamy Cauliflower & Carrot Soup

4 serving 30 minutes

Ingredients

- 2 tbsps Extra Virgin Olive Oil
- 6 stalks Green Onion (chopped)
- 5 Carrot (medium size, chopped)
- 1 head Cauliflower (chopped into florets)
- 6 cups Water
- 2 tsps Dried Thyme
- ½ tsp Sea Salt
- ½ cup Parsley

Nutrition

- Amount per serving
- Calories 137 g
- Fat 8g
- Carbs 17g
- Fiber   6g
- Sugar 7g
- Protein 4g
- Sodium406mg

Directions

1. Heat the olive oil in a large stock pot over medium-low heat. Add the green onions and saute until softened. Add the carrot, cauliflower, water, thyme and salt. Cover the pot and bring to a boil. Once boiling, reduce to a simmer. Let simmer for 20 minutes then add in the parsley and stir until wilted. Turn off the heat.

2. Puree the soup using a blender or handheld immersion blender. (Note: If using a regular blender, be careful. Ensure you leave a space for the steam to escape.) Taste and adjust seasoning if needed. Ladle into bowls and enjoy!

Notes

Make it Fancy, Roast up some leftover carrots and cauliflower and use as a garnish with pumpkin seeds.

Anti-Inflammator, Add turmeric powder.

Make it a Meal, Stir in lentils, chickpeas or chicken.

Gut-Healing, Make with bone broth instead of water. Adjust sea salt accordingly if the broth is salted.

Spicy Roasted Red Pepper Soup

4 serving 1 hour

Ingredients

- 4 Red Bell Pepper
- 1 ½ tsps. Extra Virgin Olive Oil
- 1 Sweet Onion (diced)
- 2 Garlic (cloves, minced)
- 1tsp Black Pepper (fresh ground)
- 1/8 oz Thyme Sprigs
- 1 Bay Leaf
- 3 cups Organic Vegetable Broth
- 3 tbsps Apple Cider Vinegar
- ¼ tsp Cayenne Pepper (less if you don't like it spicy)

Nutrition

- Amount per serving
- Calories 90 g
- Fat 2g
- Carbs 17g
- Fiber   4g
- Sugar 11g

- Protein 2g
- Sodium503mg

Directions

1 . Preheat oven to broil. Cut bell peppers in half lengthwise and discard seeds. Place pepper halves skin side down on a parchment paper-lined baking sheet. Broil for 15 minutes or until blackened.

2. Place roasted peppers in a zip-lock bag and seal. Let sit for 15 minutes. This allows you to peel the skin off more easily. Remove peppers from bag and peel away the skin. Throw the skin away and coarsely chop the remaining pepper.

3. Heat the oil in a large pot over medium heat. Add onion and sauté for 5 minutes or until golden. Then add garlic and sauté for another minute.

4. Add bell peppers, fresh ground pepper, bay leaf, thyme, broth, vinegar and cayenne. Bring to a boil then cover and reduce heat to simmer for 10 minutes. After 10 minutes, remove the bay leaf and thyme sprigs from the soup and discard.

5. Puree soup. You can do this with a blender, magic bullet or hand/immersion blender. If you are blending with a normal blender, ensure you remove the centerpiece of the lid to allow a place for steam to escape. Otherwise the steam will pop the lid off when blending, which is super dangerous.

6. Pour soup back into pot and warm over medium heat. Ladle into soup bowls when ready to eat. Season with a pinch of cayenne for a spicier soup. Enjoy!

Creamy Cauliflower Soup

4 serving 1 hour

Ingredients

- 1tbsp Coconut Oil
- ½ Sweet Onion (chopped)
- 1 Carrot (chopped)
- 1 head Cauliflower (cut into florets)
- 2 cups Organic Vegetable Broth
- 1 cupWater
- 1 cup Organic Coconut Milk
- ¼ tsp Sea Salt (or more to taste)
- 1 tsp   Nutmeg
- 1 Avocado (peeled and sliced)
- 2 stalks Green Onion (chopped)

Nutrition

- Amount per serving
- Calories 283 g
- Fat 22g
- Carbs 19g
- Fiber   7g
- Sugar 8g
- Protein 5g
- Sodium553mg

Directions

1. Add coconut oil to a large pot and place over medium heat. Saute the onions and carrots for about 5 minutes or until soft and golden.

2. Add the cauliflower and cook until it browns (about 5 minutes).

3. Add the broth and water. Bring to a boil. Reduce heat to simmer and cover. Let simmer for 30 minutes.

4.Add in coconut milk, sea salt and nutmeg. Stir well until milk is heated through and remove from heat.

5. With caution, puree your soup using a blender. Ensure lid is on tightly. (NOTE: If using a regular blender, ensure to remove the centerpiece of the lid and cover with a tea towel to allow a place for the steam to escape. Otherwise the steam will cause the lid to pop off, creating a mess and potentially burning yourself.)

6. Pour into bowl and top with sliced avocado and green onion. Sprinkle with fresh ground pepper and serve!

Creamy Carrot Soup

4 serving 50 minutes

Ingredients

- 1 tbsp Extra Virgin Olive Oil
- 8 Carrot (chopped into 1 inch rounds)
- 1 Sweet Onion (chopped)
- 2 Garlic (cloves, minced)
- 1 tsp Cumin
- 1 tsp Turmeric Sea Salt & Black Pepper (to taste)
- 3 cups Organic Vegetable Broth
- 1 cup Unsweetened Almond Milk
- 1 Lemon (cut into wedges)
- 1 cup Baby Spinach (chopped)

Nutrition

- Amount per serving
- Calories 133 g
- Fat 5g
- Carbs 22g
- Fiber   5g
- Sugar 11g
- Protein 3g
- Sodium629mg

Directions

1. In a large pot, heat olive oil over medium heat. Stir in onion, garlic, carrots, cumin and turmeric. Season with salt and pepper to taste. Sautee for about 10 minutes or until veggies start to brown.

2. Add in vegetable broth. Cover with lid and let simmer for 30 minutes.

3. After 30 minutes, pour in almond milk and stir well. Transfer soup to a blender to puree. Always be careful to leave a hole for the steam to escape or the lid will pop off while blending (DANGER!). Blend in batches and transfer back to pot. Taste and season with more sea salt and pepper if desired.

4. Ladle soup into bowls. Garnish with chopped spinach and drizzle with a squeeze of lemon wedge. Serve with an organic piece of bread for dipping and/or a mixed greens salad.

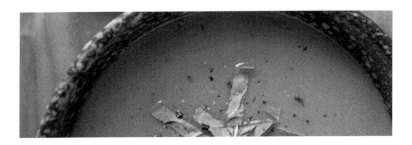

Creamy Roasted Tomato Soup

4 serving 1 hour

- **Ingredients**
- 7 Tomato (sliced into quarters)
- 2 Sweet Onion (coarsley chopped)
- 4 Garlic (cloves, peeled)
- 1 tbsp Extra Virgin Olive Oil
- 2 cups Organic Vegetable Broth
- 1 tbsp Thyme
- tsp Oregano
- 1/8 tsp Cayenne Pepper
- 1 tbsp Apple Cider Vinegar
- ½ cup Basil Leaves (chopped)
- 1 cup Unsweetened Almond Milk Sea Salt & Black Pepper (to taste)
- ½ cupBaby Spinach (chopped)

Nutrition

- Amount per serving
- Calories 136 g
- Fat 5g
- Carbs 22g
- Fiber 4g
- Sugar 9g

- Protein 5g
- Sodium466mg

Directions

1. Preheat the oven to 410°F (210°C). Toss your tomatoes, onion and garlic cloves in olive oil and season with sea salt and pepper. Place on large parchment- lined baking sheet and bake for 40 to 50 minutes.

2. In the mean time, add your vegetable broth, thyme, oregano, cayenne pepper, basil leaves and apple cider vinegar to a large stock pot. When your veggies are done roasting also add them to your stock pot. Stir in almond milk.

3. Transfer mixture to blender and blend in batches until pureed. Ensure you leave a place for the steam to escape to avoid the lid bursting off during blending.

4. Transfer pureed soup back to stock pot and warm through over low heat. Serve topped with chopped spinach and a piece of organic bread for dipping.

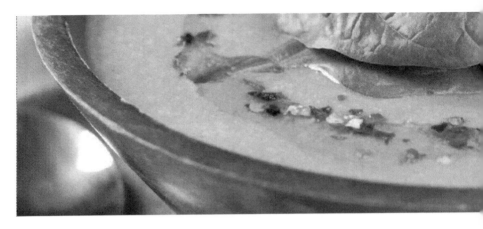

Cream of Mushroom Soup

4 serving 30 minutes

Ingredients

- 2 tbsps Coconut Oil
- 1 cup Red Onion (diced)
- 3 stalksCelery (diced)
- 2 Carrot (diced)
- 3 cups Mushrooms (any type will work)
- 1 tsp   Black Pepper
- 3 tbsps Tamari
- 4 cups Water
- ½ cup Cashews (soaked and drained)

Nutrition

Amount per serving

- Calories 214 g
- Fat 15g
- Carbs 16g
- Fiber   3g
- Sugar 6g
- Protein 7g

- Sodium811mg

Directions

1. Heat your coconut oil in a large stockpot over medium heat. Add the onion and saute for 4 - 5 minutes or until translucent. Add in the celery, carrots, mushrooms, black pepper, tamari and water. Bring to a boil and then reduce to a simmer. Cover with a lid and cook for 20 minutes.

2. Add your cashews to the blender. Ladle in one cup of your soup broth and blend well until smooth to create your cashew cream. Now ladle in the rest of your soup and puree. CAUTION: Ensure you leave a place for the steam to escape from the blender, otherwise the lid will blow off and that is bad news.

3. Ladle soup into bowls. Enjoy!

Notes

Leftovers, Refrigerate in an airtight container for up to five days. Freeze for up to two months.

Serving Size, One serving equals approximately 2 cups.

Make it Green, Add in a few handfuls of spinach or kale before blending.

Nut-Free, Use sunflower seeds instead of cashews.

Whole Mushroom Lover, Use a slotted spoon to strain out some of the mushrooms before blending, then add them back into the pureed soup.

Toppings, Top with red pepper flakes, a splash of olive oil and/or chopped baby spianch.

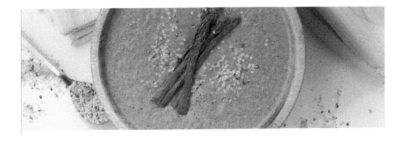

Cream of Celery & Asparagus Soup

4 serving 25 minutes

Ingredients

- 2 tbsps Coconut Oil
- 1 Yellow Onion (chopped)
- 6 stalks Celery (chopped)
- 3 Garlic (cloves, minced)
- 4 cups Water
- 1 tsp Sea Salt
- ½ tsp Black Pepper
- 3 cups Asparagus (woody ends snapped off)
- ½ cupHemp Seeds
- 4 cups Baby Spinach

Nutrition

Amount per serving

- Calories 222 g
- Fat 17g
- Carbs 12g
- Fiber   5g
- Sugar 5g
- Protein 10g
- Sodium671mg

Directions

1. Heat coconut oil in a large stock pot over medium heat. Add yellow onion and celery. Saute for 5 minutes or until veggies are slightly softened. Add minced garlic and saute for another minute.

2. Add water, sea salt and black pepper to the stock pot. Cover and bring to a boil then reduce to a simmer. Remove lid and set asparagus on top. Cover and let steam for 5 minutes or until bright green.

3. Add hemp seeds and baby spinach to your blender. Pour soup over top and puree. Ladle into bowls. Enjoy!

Notes

No Hemp Seeds, Use cashews.

Add Some Crunch, Set aside a few spears of asparagus, roast before serving and use as a garnish.

No Spinach, Use kale, swiss chard or any leafy green.

Leftovers, Store in an airtight container in the fridge for up to four days. Freeze in a freezer-safe container for up to three months.

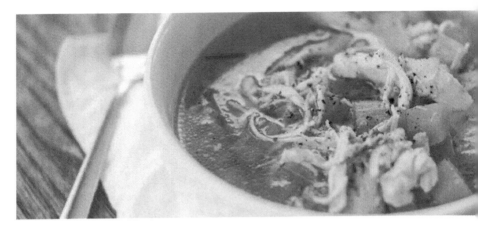

Slow Cooker Chicken Soup

6 serving 6 hours

Ingredients

- 1 Yellow Onion (diced)
- 4 stalks Celery (diced)
- 3 Carrot (medium, chopped)
- 1 tbspRosemary (fresh)
- 8ozs Chicken Breast (boneless, skinless)
- 1 Ib Chicken Thighs (boneless, skinless) Sea Salt & Black Pepper (to taste)
- 6 cups Water (or broth)

Nutrition

Amount per serving

- Calories 161 g
- Fat 4g
- Carbs 6g
- Fiber   2g
- Sugar 3g
- Protein 24g
- Sodium137mg

Directions

1. Add all ingredients to the crock pot and cook on low for 6-8 hrs.

2. Once chicken is cooked through, transfer it to a large bowl and shred it with two forks. Return the shredded chicken to the crock pot and let it soak for at least 5- 10 minutes before serving. Adjust seasoning as needed.

Notes

More carbs, Add chopped potatoes or cooked rice/pasta. You can also mix in raw pasta about 15 minutes before serving.

Leftovers, Refrigerate in an air-tight container up to 3-4 days or freeze up to 6 months. Omit pasta and potatoes if you plan to freeze.

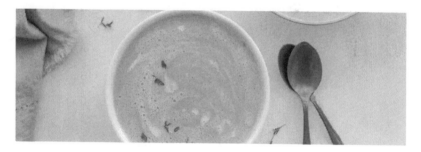

Pressure Cooker Carrot Ginger Soup

4 serving 25 minutes

Ingredients

- 3 cups Organic Vegetable Broth
- 1 Yellow Onion (chopped)
  o Garlic (clove, minced)
- 1 tbsp Ginger (fresh, minced)

- 6 Carrot (chopped)
  - o tsps Thyme (fresh, chopped)
- 1 ¼ cups Organic Coconut Milk (full fat, from a can)

Nutrition

- Amount per serving
- Calories 192 g
- Fat 14g
- Carbs 16g
- Fiber   3g
- Sugar 8g
- Protein 3g
- Sodium574mg

Directions

1. Turn the pressure cooker to sauté mode. Add a splash of vegetable broth along with the onion and cook for 3 to 4 minutes. Add the garlic and ginger and sauté for 1 minute more.

2. Turn the sauté mode off and add the carrots, thyme and rest of the broth. Put the lid on and set to "sealing" then press manual/pressure cooker and cook for 5 minutes on high pressure. Once finished, release the pressure manually.

3. Carefully remove the lid, and purée the soup using an immersion blender or a blender. Add the coconut milk and stir to combine. Serve and enjoy!

Notes

Leftovers, Refrigerate in an airtight container for up to four days. Freeze for up to three

Serving Size, One serving is equal to approximately 1 1/2 cups of soup.

Additional Toppings, Top with fresh thyme, chives or sesame seeds.

WEEKEND SOUP DETOX

Now, I'm going to keep this short and sweet, so we can get right into the recipes and meal plans.

However, before you start, here are some "best practices".

Step #1: Below you will see options for breakfast, lunch and dinner. That means we're going to stick with 3 meals a day and no snacking (not even on "healthy" foods").

If you want to kick things up a notch, you can "fast" and skip one meal (breakfast, for instance). This is 100% optional but some have seen increased results by adding in fasting.

You'll be eating protein, good fats, and veggies for breakfast and lunch, followed by soup for dinner.

Step #2: This program is based off eating healthy protein, good fats, and carbs mainly from vegetables. It's a simple formula that works 99% of the time. So even after this program is over, if you simply focus on have healthy protein, good fats, and carbs from veggies at every meal, your weight loss will continue.

Step #3: The reason this program works so well is because we're reprogramming your body to burn your stored fat for energy, instead of carbs/sugar. This is how you burn fat and lose weight without exercising.

It's very powerful, which is why we're cutting out sugars, grains, and harmful cooking oils. Going forward, please keep those 3 out of your diet as much as possible.

Alright, let's get on to the plan!

Day #1: Breakfast

Scrambled Eggs with Bacon and Spring Onions

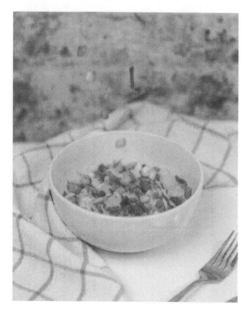

Serves 2

Cook and Prep time: 10 minutes

Ingredients:

- 4 eggs
- 2 tbsp butter
- 2 slices bacon
- 2 stalks scallions, chopped
- Salt and pepper to taste
- Hot sauce of choice if all natural(optional)

Directions

1. Melt butter in saucepan on medium high heat.
2. Add bacon, stir and cook until crispy.
3. In a small bowl, whisk eggs and pour into saucepan with bacon, stirring constantly until eggs are cooked through.
4. Add salt and pepper to taste.
5. Divide between two bowls, top with scallions (and hot sauce if using).
6. Serve immediately.

Nutrition Facts

Servings 2.0

Amount Per Serving calories 285

% Daily Value *

Total Fat 25 g   38 %

Saturated Fat 12 g   58 %

Monounsaturated Fat 8 g

Polyunsaturated Fat 3 g

Trans Fat 0 g

Cholesterol 410 mg   137 %

Sodium 304 mg   13 %

Potassium 183 mg   5 %

Total Carbohydrate 1 g0 %

Dietary Fiber 0 g   0 %

Sugars 1 g

Protein 15 g   30 %

Vitamin A   108 %

Vitamin C   0%

Calcium   9 %

Iron   11 %

*   The Percent Daily Values are based on a 2,000 calorie diet, so your values may change depending on your calorie needs. The values here may not be 100% accurate because the recipes have not been professionally evaluated nor have they been evaluated by the U.S. FDA

Day #1: Lunch

Grilled Chicken Greek Salad

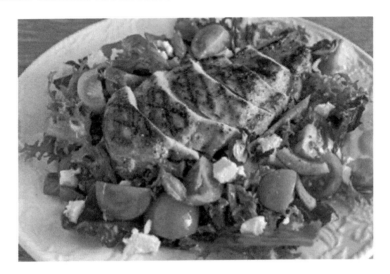

- 4 cups romaine or mixed greens
- 1 cup red leaf lettuce, torn
- 1 grilled chicken breast, sliced thin, set aside.
- 4 tbsp. feta cheese, crumbled
- 4 tbsp red onion, sliced thin

Dressing

- juice of one lemon
- 4 tbsp olive oil
- 1/2 tsp garlic powder
- 2 tbsp apple cider vinegar
- pepper to taste

Directions

1. In two bowls, add lettuce, feta, and onion. Blend lightly.
2. Lay 1/2 of sliced chicken breast on each salad.

3.   Whisk dressing ingredients in a small bowl and drizzle over each salad before serving.

Nutrition Facts

Servings 2.0

Amount Per Serving calories 422

% Daily Value *

Total Fat 33 g   51 %

Saturated Fat 7 g   36 %

Monounsaturated Fat 20 g

Polyunsaturated Fat 4 g

Trans Fat 0 g

Cholesterol 50 mg   17 %

Sodium 441 mg   18 %

Potassium 379 mg   11 %

Total Carbohydrate 12 g   4 %

Dietary Fiber 3 g   10 %

Sugars 4 g

Protein 20 g   41 %

Vitamin A   415 %

Vitamin C   42 %

Calcium   47 %

Iron   4 %

*   The Percent Daily Values are based on a 2,000 calorie diet, so your values may change depending on your calorie needs. The values here may not be 100% accurate because the recipes have not been professionally evaluated nor have they been evaluated by the U.S. FDA.

Day #1: Dinner

Italian Beefy Tomato Soup (crock-pot)

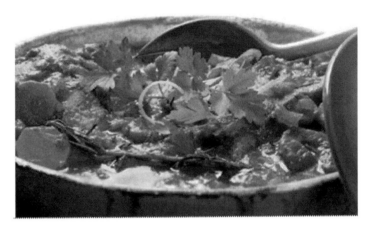

Serves 8

Cook and prep time: 15 minutes prep + 8 hours in crockpot

Ingredients

- 1 - 2 pound grass-fed beef chuck roast (pot roast)
- 3 Tbsp. apple cider vinegar

- 3 cups beef stock or broth (can use homemade, all natural or organic)
- 1 8 oz. can tomato
- 1 Tbsp. Arrowroot powder
- 3 cloves garlic diced
- 1 cup mixed mushrooms
- 2 carrots, chopped
- 1 small yellow onion sliced
- 1 tsp. dried basil
- 1 tbsp. italian parsley
- 1 1/2 tbsp. sea salt
- 1 8 oz. Can diced tomatoes in juice
- 1/2 tsp. Fresh ground pepper
- 1 large bunch of fresh italian parsley for garnish

Directions

1. Set slow cooker on low for 8 hours.
2. Add all ingredients into slow cooker except 1/2 cup of beef broth and arrowroot powder and cover. Also save fresh parsley for garnish after cooking.
3. Cook for 6 hours.
4. After 6 hours, whisk arrowroot powder with beef broth in a small bowl and blend into crock pot, stirring gently. Separate meat into large chunks with 2 forks.
5. Cook for 2 more hours.
6. Top with fresh parsley before serving.

Nutrition Facts

Servings 8.0

Amount Per Serving calories 249

% Daily Value *

Total Fat 15 g   23 %

Saturated Fat 6 g   31 %

Monounsaturated Fat 0 g

Polyunsaturated Fat 0 g

Trans Fat 0 g

Cholesterol 53 mg   18 %

Sodium 1368 mg   57 %

Potassium 383 mg   11 %

Total Carbohydrate 10 g   3 %

Dietary Fiber 4 g   17 %

Sugars 2 g

Protein 20 g   39 %

Vitamin A   67 %

Vitamin C   12 %

Calcium   27 %

Iron   58 %

*   The Percent Daily Values are based on a 2,000 calorie diet, so your values may change depending on your calorie needs. The values here may not be 100% accurate because the recipes have not been professionally evaluated nor have they been evaluated by the U.S. FDA.

Repeat this meal plan for a total of 3 days. Especially with the soup, you should have plenty for leftovers.

Printed in Great Britain
by Amazon